CW00370338

·····⋙ BHARTI VYAS'S ⋘·····
WHOLE BODY BEAUTY WISDOM

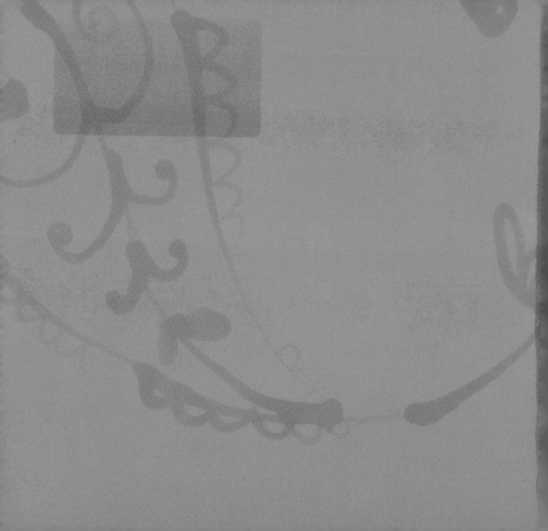

⋯⇒✤ BHARTI VYAS'S ✤⇐⋯

WHOLE BODY BEAUTY WISDOM

500 Tips for Making Your Beauty Shine Inside and Out

MARLOWE & COMPANY
NEW YORK

BHARTI VYAS'S WHOLE BODY BEAUTY WISDOM:
500 Tips for Making Your Body Shine Inside and Out

Copyright © 2005 by Bharti Vyas
Based on text written by Bhart Vyas, Jane Warren, and Clare Haggard

Published by
Marlowe & Company
An Imprint of Avalon Publishing Group Incorporated
245 West 17th Street • 11th floor
New York, NY 10011

AVALON
publishing group incorporated

Originally published in Great Britain in 2005 by Ebury Press.
This edition published by arrangement.

All rights reserved. No part of this book may be reproduced in whole or in part without written permission from the publisher, except by reviewers who may quote brief excerpts in connection with a review in a newspaper, magazine, or electronic publication; nor may any part of this book be reproduced, stored in a retrieval system, or transmitted in any form or by any means electronic, mechanical, photocopying, recording, or other, without written permission from the publisher.

Library of Congress Cataloging-in-Publication Data is Available.

ISBN: 1-56924-327-1
ISBN-13: 978-1-56924-327-5

9 8 7 6 5 4 3 2 1

Printed in China

CONTENTS

INTRODUCTION
BY BHARTI VYAS

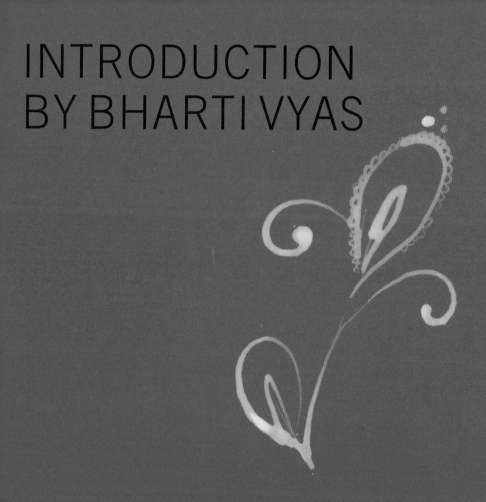

I have written this book because I strongly believe that everyone has the right to look and feel good. Beauty does not solely belong to those who can afford it. In this book, you will discover the knowledge that will enable you to take control of your own health, beauty and well-being at a minimal cost. I have put together some of the best practical tips, so that you can initiate a tailor-made home therapy system that works specifically for you. This book will also help you to ask the right questions if you should go to a beauty salon in search of true therapy.

So where do these tips come from? They come from my 25 years' experience as a practicing holistic beauty therapist and many have been drawn from my childhood and my Indian culture. As a child, my parents and grandparents used Ayurvedic principles to treat many minor health and beauty problems. These natural and simple applications can make a profound difference to our mind, body, and soul. And now I hand these tips on to you. My philosophy has always been that "beauty on the outside . . .

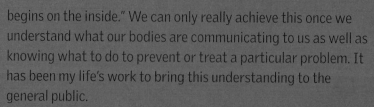

begins on the inside." We can only really achieve this once we understand what our bodies are communicating to us as well as knowing what to do to prevent or treat a particular problem. It has been my life's work to bring this understanding to the general public.

With this in mind, I developed the BVM (Bharti Vyas Method). It integrates all my knowledge and experiences into one simple method that envelops everything we need to maintain good health and a sense of prolonged well-being, while looking and feeling beautiful in the process.

The BVM is threefold: salon therapy, home therapy, and diet and lifestyle. It is based on knowledge and understanding of how the body works, combined with the practical know-how on how to rebalance it. The BVM draws together a myriad of worldwide therapies that are combined with the latest technology. It incorporates the principles of Ayurveda, acupressure, magnet therapy, and lymphatic drainage and various massage techniques alongside the BV Ultimate Therapy Range of treatments. These aspects work synergistically to help balance the mind, body, and soul. Many salons nationally and internationally are now using the BVM successfully to help their clients maintain long-term vitality and health.

Bharti Vyas's Whole Body Beauty Wisdom is a great starting point for changing the way you look and feel. Make it part of your lifestyle and looking after your beauty and well-being will come naturally, not only for you but your whole family.

Bharti Vyas

OUTER HEALTH

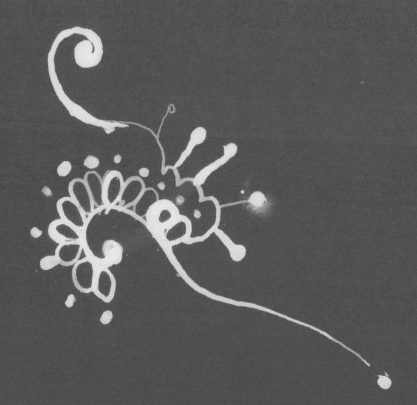

In our busy modern lives, many of us require superhuman stamina to do all that is demanded of us—to bring up a family and keep the various elements of a household running smoothly, often at the same time as holding down a job. Our health and well-being are therefore a top priority—hence the importance of looking after ourselves. If we don't make a point of it no-one else will.

FACE

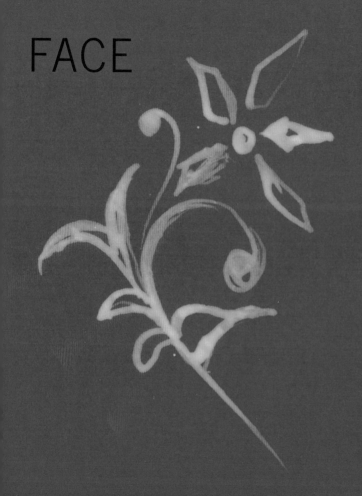

CLEANSING

It may seem like an obvious point, but keeping your skin clean is the number-one skincare priority. You need to cleanse your face both night and morning: in the morning to remove surface oil and dead skin cells after the night-time repair work to the skin has taken place, so that you begin the day with fresh skin; in the evenings to remove the grime that has accumulated during the day and all traces of make-up. The morning routine need be no more than a swipe with a damp face cloth, but the evening cleanse should be extremely thorough. Any residue left on the skin slows down the repair process of the tissue and prevents the skin from "breathing." Remember: for cleansing purposes, your face starts at your collarbone and stops at your hairline.

✲ To cleanse your nose properly, you need to cover the sides, stem, grooves, and tip. If the skin on your nose is oily or congested, wrap a flannel around your index finger, lubricate it with a mild soap, oatmeal scrub (see page 84) or a mild commercial exfoliant and, using small circular movements, go over the entire nose twice.

✲ One of the oldest and gentlest methods of cleansing the skin is oil; it is particularly good for mature skins. Apply a light film of almond or sunflower oil all over your neck and face (including your eyelids) and rub in gently. Leave for up to a minute and remove with dampened cotton wool or a facial sponge.

secret quick cleanser

If you are short of time and require an extra radiance boost, try this super-quick cleansing technique:

Pour boiling water into a basin over the juice of half a lemon and a splash of rosewater—add real rose petals if you have them to hand.

Hold your face over the steam with a towel to trap the vapors, breathe deeply and pat dry afterward.

This is a wonderful cleanser that keeps your skin fresh and also invigorates you internally.

TONING

As the name suggests, toners have a mild (and short-lived) tightening effect on the skin. They are also great skin refreshers. Toners with a significant proportion of alcohol are described as astringents and should only be used on oily skins because of their drying action. They also have valuable antiseptic properties.

Rosewater makes a freshening and fragrant tonic for dry and sensitive skin types.

Witch hazel mixed with a little water or saline solution is an effective toner. Use a very small proportion of witch hazel on older skins, as it can have a drying effect.

One of the best natural toners is cold water. This can be splashed lightly onto your face—even your eyes—and directed at other parts of your body using a shower head, to bring fresh blood to the surface.

MOISTURIZING

Our skin is equipped with its own natural moisturizer, a combination of sebum and sweat excreted all over the surface of our bodies via our follicles and pores. Moisturizing creams, which are basically oil and water emulsions, are based on the same ingredients, combined in varying proportions to create lighter or richer formulations. They should operate on the same natural principle, supporting this natural process and making up for any deficiencies.

FACT
THE TENDENCY TO OVER-MOISTURIZE UNDERMINES
THE SKIN'S CAPACITY TO KEEP ITSELF TAUT. ALLOW
YOURSELF TO BE GUIDED BY THE CHANGING CONDITION
OF YOUR SKIN—AND DON'T BE AFRAID TO LEAVE
IT BARE OCCASIONALLY.

The basic function of a moisturizer is to maintain softness by keeping up the water level in the outermost layer of skin cells. It does this by creating a watertight seal that prevents what would otherwise be the continuous process of evaporation from the surface. At the same time, it provides a buffer to keep out potential "invaders," thereby safeguarding the health of the lower regions of the skin, and ultimately the inner body.

❊ Use a light, oil-free moisturizer that will leave a protective film on the skin. Choose a non-comedogenic formulation, i.e. one that will not block pores.

❊ Get into the habit of applying oil or cream to slightly damp skin—night and morning—as this helps to "lock in" valuable extra moisture.

❊ A layer of moisturizer creates a good base for and a barrier against make-up. Leave for 10 minutes and tissue off excess before applying foundation.

❊ If you are wearing separate sunscreen, apply it after your moisturizer, at least 15 minutes before going out into the sun.

EXFOLIATION

For our skin to remain clear, smooth, and translucent, the surface layer needs to be kept free of any superfluous cells and its excretory activities able to continue unimpeded. That is why we exfoliate—to buff away the dead cells that might otherwise clog our pores and dull our complexion. The very act of removing this redundant top layer appears to stimulate cell reproduction lower down in the epidermis—an increasing concern as our skin begins to age. Although any skin will benefit from gentle exfoliation once a week to refine the texture and clear the pores, take care: overenthusiastic exfoliation can undermine the barrier function of the skin and may even damage the underlying tissue.

For a physical exfoliator or scrub, choose between a shop-bought product or a homemade preparation using a natural exfoliator such as oatmeal (see page 83).

When you exfoliate, apply the paste to damp skin and rub very lightly using circular movements. Ensure you stroke rather than scour, and moisturize your skin well afterward.

Newly exfoliated skin is more vulnerable to sun damage so apply a sun block if you are going out in the sun.

SUNCARE

Shielding the skin from sun damage from earliest infancy is the surest way to protect the skin and avoid wrinkles. Keep out of the sun as much as possible and wear a hat to protect both your face and hair.

Antioxidant vitamins A, C and E—either in tablet form or applied to your face at night in an oil or cosmetic cream formulation—will help to limit damage by the sun's rays.

There is no better insurance policy against sun damage than an application of SPF 15 cream every day of the year.

recommended
skincare essentials:

Exfoliating cleanser to "polish" the side of your neck and face

Therapeutic oils to nourish the underlying tissues

Moisturizing cream with a high UV factor (at least SPF 15)
to protect your skin from sun damage

Rich moisturizer to bolster your skin in harsh winter weather

Moisturizing lotion for your body

Dead Sea salts for your bath (see page 76).

EYES

One of our most beautiful and individual features, our eyes reflect our vitality, emotions, and general state of health. How we use them is also important: bright eyes and immediate eye contact impart directness and confidence; downcast eyes suggest timidity and low self-esteem.

Despite the faith placed in cosmetic eye creams, the surest way to nourish the skin and look after the health of your eyes is by eating well and by giving the circulation a regular helping hand. Eyes also flourish on a simple regime of rest, exercise, and natural light. They do not respond well to excessive smoking or alcohol.

Take care not to pull or drag the skin around the eyes when applying or removing make-up as this can hasten the arrival of premature wrinkles.

The underlying tissue around the eyes is poorly supplied with sebaceous glands, so the eye area needs good lubrication and nourishment. The surest way to nourish the skin is by eating well and by giving the circulation a regular helping hand with light massage (see page 99).

Soothe your eyes: place a slice of cucumber on each eyelid for up to 15 minutes. Cucumber's high mineral and water content is therapeutic for the eyes, and the juice makes a nourishing eye drop.

❋ Always wear sunglasses (with ultraviolet or UV and infrared ray protection) in bright sunlight. Your eyes do need natural light but make sure they are unshaded only in gentle sunlight.

❋ For firm, taut eyelids: shut both eyelids tightly so that you feel the squeezing effect on the eyes. Maintain this pressure for a count of 12. Relax the eyelids. Rest the eyes for a moment by keeping them lightly closed. Repeat five times.

❋ To keep your eyes white and bright, apply cold milk to your eyelids with cotton wool each morning like a toner.

❋ Use the bare minimum of products on your eyes—stick to natural products only.

✂ Never use a toner on the eyes: simply splash your eyes with cold water after cleansing, which will also invigorate the circulation.

✂ Don't fall into the trap of slathering your eyes with a super-rich cream to replace lost moisture and restore suppleness, as this will simply overtax the delicate eye tissue and do nothing to enhance your eyes.

✂ To create a natural and flattering eyebrow shape, start by removing hairs from the inner edge and the bridge of the nose. Now prune the center and outer edge, allowing the line to taper gradually to nothing. To find out where the brow should end, imagine a line connecting the outside of your nostril with the outer corner of your eye and extending out to your brow. Finally pull out any stray hairs below the brows.

LIPS

Our mouth is the most sensual feature of our face, both from the point of view of our appearance and the sensations it enables us to experience. The texture and condition of our lips contribute as much as the overall shape and contours of our mouth to its allure. A deft hand with the right lipstick and a healthy set of teeth are all that is required to complete the picture.

Twitching your nose is an effective way of mobilizing the muscles in the middle of the face: make small up-and-down movements without creating too many creases over the bridge. This activates the skin between the nose and mouth.

Almond oil applied to your lips and the skin around your mouth will help to keep the area supple.

If you smoke, stop now! Pucker lines and wrinkles on the upper lip come early to heavy smokers, due to the repeated movements of the mouth involved in the very action of smoking.

facial exercises
for the mouth

**Do this exercise whenever you have a spare moment
and you could feel a firming effect in as little as a week.**

Close your mouth and inflate the skin above the upper
lip and on either side of the mouth, while you continue
to breathe through your nose.

Hold for a count of 10 and then repeat 10 times.
Keep your upper lip smooth and relaxed throughout—
it may help to position one finger above each corner
of your mouth to hold the skin in place.

- Face cloths are very useful for sweeping away dead skin cells in the area above the lip—they will also ginger up the circulation without subjecting your skin to further irritation.

- To boost the circulation and lift dead skin, massage your lips from time to time with a soft toothbrush.

- Don't be afraid to use lipstick—it's an important tool and an increasingly valuable prop as we age. See pages 228–30 for tips on applying lipstick.

TEETH AND GUMS

The importance of oral hygiene cannot be overemphasized. Unless you protect your teeth and gums with regular and effective brushing and flossing, you are inviting decay and gum disease. Eventually this may mean the loss of teeth and the erosion of underlying tissue and bone.

❊ Ensure you are using a toothpaste that contains fluoride—
and schedule a dental check-up every six months.

❊ Floss between all your teeth several times a week and brush
your teeth at least twice a day.

❊ Massage your gums by brushing them with your toothbrush.
If they bleed, it is a sure sign that they are unhealthy, in which
case you should redouble your efforts.

❊ To build and maintain strong teeth, make sure you have
an adequate intake of calcium and vitamins C and D.

Gargle every day with a few mouthfuls of warm salt water to keep germs and infections at bay (a generous pinch of salt to half a glass of water).

Invigorate your gums with a salt rub, which will leave your mouth feeling thoroughly refreshed.

To whiten teeth, use bicarbonate of soda on a damp toothbrush and polish until they gleam. Remember, however, that white teeth do not exist—teeth are all variations on a shade of cream.

JAWLINE AND CHIN

A smooth, slender jawline undoubtedly contributes to an impression of leanness throughout the face, although razor-sharp definition can be harsh and unbecoming. A fleshy jawline, however, blurs the definition of the face and, rightly or wrongly, often signals "fat."

❧ By massaging along your jawline, you can prevent stagnation occurring and release a lot of the tension held in this part of the face, which can otherwise lead to headaches and dental problems.

❧ To keep your jawline in trim, rest one elbow on a firm surface and cup your chin in the palm of your hand. Push your chin into the palm, which should resist the pressure. Hold for a slow count of five. Repeat five times.

NECK

The neck is one of the most naturally graceful—
and hard-working—parts of the body. A supple
neck makes for a youthful and vivacious appearance.
Indeed, the lively head movements of a young
person are in many ways a perfect definition
of natural beauty.

⟮⟯ To release and realign your neck and shoulders, imagine that your head is being pulled upward by a piece of string attached to the crown.

⟮⟯ If you use a VDU (Visual Display Unit) raise the height of it, so that your neck is not permanently inclined as you look at it. Also make a point of holding reading material up before your eyes rather than bending your neck to read it on a flat surface.

⟮⟯ Cleanse your neck night and morning in the same way as your face, starting at the collarbones and working up to the jawline.

⟮⟯ Apply a rich moisturizing cream to your neck at night, and a moisturizer combined with sunscreen during the day. Do not forget to include the sides of your neck and the area around your collarbones.

the Lion pose

The following exercise performed once a day will stop your face and neck muscles from ever going into retirement.

Take a deep breath and, as you breathe out slowly, open your mouth as wide as possible and stick your tongue out as far as it will go. At the same time, look at the ceiling without raising your head or straining your eyes.

Maintain the position and count slowly up to 12. Aim for five repetitions.

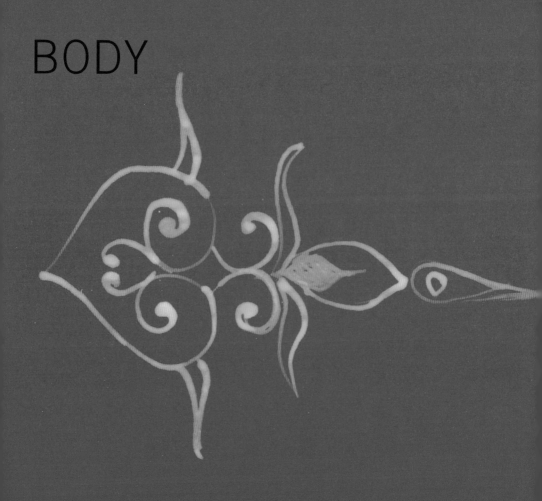

BODY

ARMS

There is something particularly attractive about a lean, well-toned upper arm. It gives the impression of a healthy, active body. By contrast, flabby, flaccid arms suggest sluggishness and inertia. Since the muscles of the upper arms move the forearms and bear most of the load when you are lifting an object, there are plenty of opportunities to put these muscles to work, without having to make a trip to the local gym.

✳ Massage your upper arms regularly with almond or olive oil for smooth, supple skin.

✳ To build long, lean biceps and triceps, raise your arms in line with your shoulder, with your palms facing down. Make a fist, squeeze and hold for a count of ten. Release and repeat five times.

✳ Take a bath in Dead Sea salts (see page 76). This will provide instant relief and therapy for overworked muscles, troublesome joints, and fluid retention in the arms, as well as restoring the skin to peachy softness.

HANDCARE

Graceful hands and beautiful nails are much-prized physical attributes. Supple hands and trim, healthy nails speak volumes about our state of health and personal grooming. Neglected hands rather let the side down. And they don't just create a poor impression—they can belie our age.

To protect your hands and nails, always wear gloves for household tasks that involve immersing your hands in water, for gardening, and in cold weather.

For graceful, silky hands use a heavy barrier cream to help protect the skin from dehydration. Keep a supply beside every sink in your home.

Apply handcream whenever your hands have come into contact with water and always last-thing at night—glycerine-based hand creams are non-greasy and help to rehydrate the skin.

In the summer, add a layer of sunscreen to your hands or look for a hand cream with built-in SPF.

mini therapy

Every time you use hand cream give your hands a mini-therapy:

Rub cream into your knuckles and finger joints using small circular movements, followed by a pulling motion to ease the joints.

Now use your thumbs to massage the backs of the hands upward in the direction of the wrist to clear any congestion.

NAILCARE

Like hair, nails consist of modified skin cells and they flourish on a similar regime to your hair. They benefit from a well-balanced diet, packed with vitamins and minerals, and an adequate supply of proteins. As we age, our nails become thicker and more brittle, and less able to retain moisture—the good habits that help you preserve your hands will also protect your nails.

Unless your nails are in mint condition, wear them no longer than the tips of your fingers, to keep them manageable. Squareish ends and straight sides look modern and practical.

Apply a nourishing cream or oil to your nails every night before you go to bed. Almond oil is a particularly good nail food and will soak easily into your hands if applied just after a bath.

File nails regularly with a large emery board, using the rough side to shorten and the smooth side to shape. Work upward in one direction rather than "sawing," as friction weakens the nails, causing them to split.

Nails and hands benefit from weekly exfoliation (try the All-Purpose Oatmeal Scrub, page 84) to smooth the surface and encourage regeneration of new cells.

routine for healthy nail growth

The frictional heat that is generated in this routine improves the flow of blood to the nail bed, assuring the delivery of nutrients and oxygen essential for strong, healthy nail growth.

Bend the fingers of both hands in toward the palms and press the nails together. Keeping your hands relaxed, rub the two sets of fingernails against one another for one minute—your thumbs will be a bit hit and miss.

Repeat this process regularly. Even if poor nail condition is a result of an underlying medical condition, more efficient circulation can assist the nourishing and repairing process.

BUST

A great deal of anxiety surrounds the whole issue of breast size and shape, and myths abound about how it is possible to make the bust more voluptuous. The proportion of fat cells—which is what makes breast size vary—is dictated by hereditary factors, weight and the natural shape of our body and can only be increased by a good diet.

❧ An easy way to create a beautiful bustline is by improving your posture. This lifts the ribcage naturally upward and outward and makes the breasts sit a little prouder on the chest.

❧ Moisturize the fine skin on your breasts regularly. Using the palms of your hands, apply almond oil or body lotion, moving upward around the breast, lifting each one gently so that you can massage the underside, and sweeping up into your armpits. This helps to clear toxins from the breast tissue while assisting the firming process.

bust toning exercise

Stretch your arms out in front of you, bend them at the elbow and grasp each forearm firmly below the elbow with the opposite hand.

Breathe in slowly through the nose and, as you breathe out, tighten your grip and hold for a count of five, increasing to ten. Repeat 10 times.

BUTTOCKS AND LEGS

It's well worth making the effort to do massage and undertake regular exercise in order to get a pair of firm, nicely rounded buttocks—they can really enhance the figure. Smooth, firm legs are not solely the preserve of models and exercise fanatics— you can make a real difference in simple ways.

✻ You will be amazed at the toning effect of regular buttock-clenching. Get into the habit of tightening your buttocks, whether standing or sitting, every time you think of it.

✻ Walk regularly to keep calf and thigh muscles active. It helps with the difficult task of pumping your blood and lymph back up the legs—this guarantees good lymphatic clearance and wards off varicose veins.

✻ When you are walking, be conscious at every step of your upper and lower leg muscles working all the time. Land on your heel and spring from one foot to the other. Squeeze your buttock muscles to propel yourself forward. This will naturally tone your legs.

two exercises for firmer thighs

Use the plié, a classic ballet posture, to work the muscles of the thighs. Place your hands on your hips and stand with your heels together and your toes pointing outward. Breathe in and rise up onto your toes. Breathe out and lower yourself into a squatting position, making sure that your back is straight. Do not go any lower than is comfortable. Breathe in again and, pressing on the balls of your feet, raise yourself as slowly as you can to the standing position. Breathe out and rest. Repeat three times.

Sit with your back up against a firm surface, your knees bent and your fingertips resting on the floor beside you. Place a cushion between your knees, breathe in and, as you breathe out, squeeze the cushion between your inner thighs for a slow count of eight. Repeat five times. Make sure your inner thighs are doing the work while other parts of your legs are relaxed.

FEET

"Out of sight is out of mind" seems to best describe
our relationship with our feet. Our feet are designed for
the unglamorous task of bearing our load, which seems
to give them a status inferior even to our hands. Given
their long years of hard service, they ought instead
to be pampered at every available opportunity.

Exfoliate your feet as often as you need to using an abrasive scrub. This will refine the skin and disperse any stagnated pigmentation around joints and other pressure points.

Stick to natural fibers on your feet and expose feet to the air for a short period every day. Go barefoot whenever you can.

Stimulate the circulation to the small joints in the toes by massaging each of your toes between your index finger and thumb. Continue for one to two minutes per toe.

Spread and wiggle toes in the bath to liven up inert feet. Make sure you always dry toes thoroughly to avoid infection.

Nourish the skin on your feet after a bath using a good anti-bacterial and anti-fungal foot cream or almond oil. This will help corns and calluses and also improve your foot hygiene.

Clip and file toenails squarely, in line with the ends of the toes, so that the growth does not head into the surrounding soft tissue.

the "foot facial"

There's no reason why you shouldn't give your feet the equivalent of a facial to keep them looking, feeling (and smelling!) good. At my clinic we give clients a "foot facial," which not only makes the feet and nails look immaculate but also boosts health and well-being. Although you won't get the same intensity of treatment at home, you can duplicate some of the effects using very simple methods.

Using Dead Sea salts (see page 76) give your feet a really intensive massage, massaging the soles, heels, toes, in between the toes, the ankle, and right up to the knee. This will help to drain trapped toxins and relieve tense muscles.

Once you have rinsed your feet, soak them in warm water. Using a cuticle pusher, push back the skin around your toenails. You can also use a pumice stone to grate off dead skin on the soles of your feet.

Rub your feet with orange oil; its sweating action helps to release toxins in congested skin, and it helps in cell regeneration. Tea tree oil has antiseptic and bactericide properties which can help ease fungal infections like athlete's foot.

HAIR AND SCALP

Our hair has the power to lift or depress our spirits. Beautiful hair is as much a source of pride for a man as it is for a woman and we spend millions of pounds teasing and taming our crowning glory in an attempt to make the most of what we've got. Yet the real secret lies in understanding how to nurture our hair and improve its condition from the inside.

Poor circulation to the scalp is at the root of many hair problems. In order to have a healthy head of hair, the tens of thousands of follicles crammed into this thick covering of skin need to be properly nourished. Good blood flow and brisk lymphatic circulation to and from your scalp "feed" hair and prevent toxic build-up.

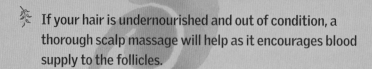

If your hair is undernourished and out of condition, a thorough scalp massage will help as it encourages blood supply to the follicles.

Massage your scalp at least once a week when you are due to wash your hair.

When you massage your scalp, the natural oils are spread evenly along the hair instead of remaining at the roots, which will make your hair look shiny, healthy, and lustrous.

❋ As well as improving the condition of your hair, a scalp massage will clear your head, lift your spirits, and evaporate stores of tension.

❋ Coconut oil is ideal for hair massage—the invisible coating left after washing acts as a protective shield, locking moisture into the hair shaft as well as providing a barrier against the sun.

❋ Buy coconut oil from pharmacies and Asian food stores—liquefy it by standing the container in a bowl of boiling water for 10–15 minutes, or microwave for one minute.

bharti's scalp massage

Measure 3 tablespoons of liquefied coconut oil into a bowl.
Dip a cotton wool into the oil and squeeze so that it's not
dripping. Apply to your hair along the central parting. Continue
to part your hair at regular intervals across the front of your
head until you reach the tips of your ears, rubbing the oil
onto the scalp as you go. Replenish the cotton wool with oil
as needed and repeat the process at the back of your head,
until every inch of your scalp is covered lightly.

Use the balls of your fingers to manipulate your scalp and help
loosen it. Apply as much pressure as is comfortable. Start gently,
pressing lightly with the fingers, progressively increasing the
pressure so that the fingers are really working the scalp. It may
take a few weeks before your scalp really starts to relax.

Pay proper attention to the section at the base of the skull by circling your thumbs along the hairline with your fingers resting on the back of your head. Pour any remaining oil onto the central parting and rub vigorously. Run your fingers through your hair to disperse the oil.

Leave the oil on for a couple of hours—overnight if possible. Problem scalps should be treated once a day for 12–14 weeks, decreasing to two or three times a week. After six months you can embark on a maintenance program of weekly treatments.

🌿 Once your scalp is in peak condition, you should only need to wash your hair twice a week.

🌿 If you want to dye your hair, try a temporary or semi-permanent color first—then you can experiment without being stuck for too long with the result.

🌿 For naturally healthy-looking hair, eat lots of fresh fruit and vegetables (raw whenever possible), eat plenty of wholegrains and dried fruits, drink eight to ten glasses of fresh water daily, and limit your intake of refined carbohydrates, saturated fats, coffee, tea, sugar, and salt.

🐝 Detangle your hair before you wash it—wet hair is extremely fragile.

🐝 Always use a gentle, pH-balanced shampoo to preserve the hair's natural acid mantle.

🐝 Squeeze shampoo into your palms before applying to your scalp and the roots of your hair—massage your scalp lightly with your fingertips, moving from the hairline toward the center—then rinse and rinse until your hair "squeaks" for a thorough hair-wash.

🐝 Use only a tiny amount of conditioner and comb it through your hair gently with a wide-toothed comb, starting at the ends and working slowly upward—then rinse, rinse, and rinse again.

Do not rub your hair—pat and squeeze it dry.

Wait until your hair is at least half-dry before attempting to style it.

Allow your hair to dry naturally as often as possible, using your hands to create shape and lift the roots.

Wash your brushes and combs regularly with shampoo or detergent.

※ Avoid hairbrushes with synthetic bristles.

※ Protect your hair from the sun—either oil your hair at least once a week, or cover your hair in intense sunlight, particularly if it is colored.

※ Wear a close-fitting cap when swimming in a chlorinated pool. Colored hair should also be protected from sea water.

※ Zinc oxide in shampoo formulations acts as a useful three-way sunscreen, conditioner, and anti-dandruff agent.

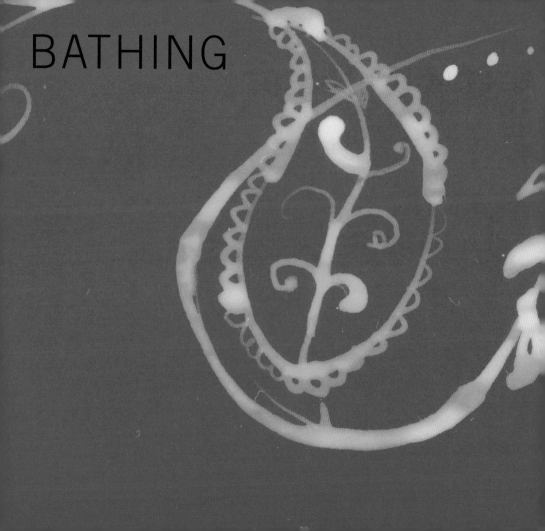

BATHING

BATH THERAPY

One of the most therapeutic treatments we can give ourselves is a long, relaxed soak in the bath. Children are also exposed to different kinds of stress and, if you teach them how to dispel such tension, you will be equipping them with a valuable means of self-protection and survival for later in life.

- Give yourself at least 30 minutes in the bath, once or twice a week.

- Make sure your bathroom is tidy and uncluttered before you have a bath—a messy room will be a distraction and you will not be able to relax fully.

- Light candles around the bathroom to evoke a relaxing atmosphere— the gentle, flickering light is more restful to the eyes than an electric bulb.

- Polish the skin on your body once weekly, either using an Oatmeal scrub (see page 84) or a mild commercial exfoliant.

⟡ Ensure your bath water is pleasantly warm—if it is too hot,
it will stimulate rather than relax your system and can have
a dehydrating and slackening effect on the skin, as well as
damaging fragile capillaries.

⟡ Add five drops of lavender oil to your bath water. It has
a soothing aroma and will help to ease aches and pains.

⟡ A few drops of sandalwood oil in your bath water will help
to dispel nervous tension, lift depression, and relieve insomnia.
It is well suited to dry skins.

dead sea salts

The very high concentration of minerals in Dead Sea salts has a natural therapeutic action on the skin and benefits the body as a whole. The effect of these minerals on the external body is to boost the skin's excretory function by dissolving the dehydrated dead cells that accumulate on the surface. This speeds up the elimination of the body's waste and has a smoothing and refining effect on the skin.

Of the 28 naturally occurring minerals in the salts, three are particularly valuable for our internal health: potassium, which regulates the fluid balance within our bodies and the circulation of blood and lymph; magnesium, our body's main "nerve food;" and bromide, which has a calming and restorative effect on the system. Because these substances are part of the body's own make-up they are immediately "recognized," absorbed, and put to use.

Regular salt baths can correct all sorts of imbalances within the body. They encourage gentle detoxification of the system and reduce fluid retention in the tissues, which can assist weight loss and relieve problems affecting the joints. They act as an antidote to the potentially damaging effects of stress and strengthen our resistance to disease. They also safeguard that cornerstone of our health and well-being: sleep. By quelling anxiety and restoring calm, a salt bath taken at the end of a gruelling day both aids and enhances sleep.

KITCHEN CUPBOARD TREATMENTS

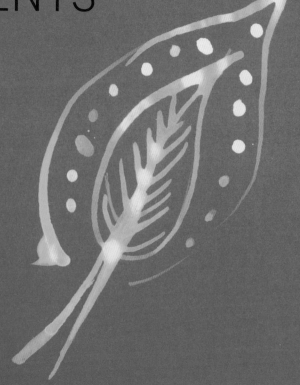

HOME REMEDIES

You don't have to spend a fortune on expensive beauty treatments and facials. Many basic cupboard ingredients are as good as, if not better than, fancy store-bought concoctions. Here are some essential tips and recipes using ingredients as simple and natural as oatmeal, lemon juice, honey, and salt.

If you feel the tell-tale tingling sensation of a cold sore, hold an ice compress against the area. Once the sore has erupted, dab on lemon juice mixed with a pinch of salt.

Honey is good for dislodging dead skin cells—it also has soothing, healing, emollient, and mildly antiseptic properties.

For dry, irritated, and sensitive skins, oats and oatflakes have a gentle but deep cleansing action and can correct skin imbalances.

Double cream has a composition not unlike a rich moisturizer, and is naturally well endowed with vitamin A, as well as useful amounts of vitamins D and E—a natural skin food.

❋ Lemon juice is a great cleanser and healer with anti-bacterial properties. A useful natural bleaching agent, it also helps to restore the skin's acid balance.

❋ Salt is a powerful cleanser and neutralizer of bacteria, as well as a natural exfoliator.

❋ The healing powers of turmeric are well known in India, where it is sprinkled onto cuts to speed up the clotting and repair process.

RECIPES

Here are some instant recipes for traditional cosmetic preparations using basic cooking ingredients. Apply masks to cleansed skin and remove immediately if you feel any discomfort. Rinse off with warm water and pat skin dry. Moisturize well afterward. The quantities given are enough for one thick application.

GENTLE FACIAL EXFOLIATOR (SENSITIVE SKIN)

2 heaping teaspoons fine oatmeal
2 teaspoons double cream

Combine ingredients, apply to skin, and rub with a very light action using the balls of your fingers, then rinse off. Do not apply sustained pressure to any particular blemish.

CLEANSING MASK (CONGESTED SKIN)

2 heaping teaspoons gram flour
1 teaspoon water
1 teaspoon honey

Mix to a thick, sticky consistency. Apply to affected areas and leave for 5–7 minutes.

ALL-PURPOSE OATMEAL SCRUB

2 tablespoons finely ground oatmeal
1 tablespoon almond oil

Combine ingredients. Also suitable for all-over body use.

STABILIZING FACE MASK (SENSITIVE SKIN, ACNE ROSACEA, PREMATURE WRINKLES)

1 heaped teaspoon gram flour
1 teaspoon double cream
2 teaspoons water and a pinch of salt

Mix to a thick and creamy consistency. Apply to skin and leave for 10 minutes before rinsing off.

HEALING MASK

2 teaspoons honey
¼ teaspoon fine sea salt
1 teaspoon turmeric

Mix to a thick paste. Apply to pimples every evening and leave on for up to 30 minutes or even overnight. Once the skin has cleared, this treatment can be used preventatively as a face pack once a month.

EYE MASK

2 teaspoons grated cucumber
1 teaspoon powdered milk

Mix to a thick paste. Close eyes and cover upper and lower eyelids. Leave for 10 minutes then wipe off with moist cotton wool.

FIRMING MASK (PUDGY, DROOPY CHEEKS)

2 heaped teaspoons gram flour
2 teaspoons water
½ teaspoon honey

Mix to a creamy paste. Leave on for 15 minutes.

LEMON-BASED MASK (EXCESS HAIR)

1 teaspoon lemon juice
1 teaspoon honey

This should be a very liquid consistency. Smooth the paste on in the direction of hair growth and leave for 10 minutes.

ECZEMA MASK

2 teaspoons gram flour
2 teaspoons almond oil
¼ teaspoon salt

This should be a smooth and fairly liquid consistency. Apply to affected area and leave for 10 minutes.

NOURISHING CHEEK MASK (COMBINATION SKIN)

2 teaspoons gram flour
2 teaspoons honey

Gooey consistency. Spread the paste over your cheeks and leave for 10 minutes.

NOSE MASK

$1/2$ teaspoon gram flour
$1/2$ teaspoon honey
a pinch of salt
a few drops of lemon juice

Cover your nose with the paste, allowing it to overlap onto your cheeks. Leave for 5–10 minutes.

AVOCADO STONE MASK

1 avocado stone
2 teaspoons yogurt

Grate the avocado stone and watch it turn from white to red.
Add a little yogurt and apply it to your face with your fingers
to polish the skin.

MASSAGE

Massage used to be the privilege of the rich and is still regarded as something of a luxury. Traditionally, wealthy people would employ masseurs to assist in the task of preserving their youthful appearance by giving their system a "cleansing" work-out. But you can apply the basic techniques of massage on your own body, to ensure that your skin is nourished properly by regulating the blood supply to the cells, and guard against stagnation and toxic build-up by assisting the process of lymphatic drainage—both essential steps in the quest for firm, clear, young-looking skin.

Set aside an hour a week to massage the key areas of your face and body—give it six weeks, and you'll start noticing a difference not just in your complexion and the texture of your skin, but in the way that you feel.

Regular massage is important for our joints, helping to relieve congestion and disperse waste that could, over time, cause deterioration and reduced mobility.

Massage transforms the condition of all skin types and increases the capacity of dry skin to absorb nourishment.

Your hands are highly sensitive and powerful beauty tools, with the ability to influence the workings of your internal body and, therefore, the health of your skin. Learn how to use your hands properly (see overleaf).

how to use your hands

Finger ball: The balls of the fingers are richly supplied with nerve endings and therefore capable of detecting any change in the skin's texture, as well as in the muscles and tissue beneath. Stimulate nerve endings and galvanize the body's blood and lymph systems into action by using small circular movements in a specified area. Apply pressure only to a depth that feels comfortable.

Palming: The palms of the hands contain many nerve junctions that radiate a lot of heat. A stroking action is useful on swollen joints and areas of the body that cannot take vigorous stimulation. Gentle, repeated palming for several minutes can trigger off the parasympathetic nervous system (i.e. not under voluntary control of the brain), which redresses the balance within the body.

Pinching: Small pinches use the thumb and index finger to work a small area such as the forehead. Large pinches require all four fingers plus the thumb and are useful for larger muscles. Pinching is a fast action that activates the nerve endings in the skin. The brain responds to the mild pain sensation by increasing circulatory activity, reviving the cells, and helping to siphon off waste via the lymph.

(•: Choose an hour on either a weekend morning or evening
to devote to your massage—you are less likely to be rushed
and stressed.

(•: Start or finish your massage routine with a good soak in the bath.

(•: Before you begin your massage routine, make sure you have
a bath mat to rest your feet on, an upright chair for best sitting
posture, cotton wool, a towel, and a glass of water to sip.

(•: Avoid using a mirror during your self-massage—it is distracting,
and if you can't see what you're doing, you're more likely to rely
on your sense of touch, which will in turn become more acute.

(•: Sitting upright while you massage yourself is important—you
need to breathe slowly and deeply throughout, which will help
to keep your muscles relaxed.

- Use oil in massage to encourage a smooth, rhythmic action and to avoid dragging the skin.

- Soak a cotton wool ball with massage oil and wipe it over the area you are going to work on—use a little more if your skin is dry.

- Set aside 30 minutes of your massage routine for facial therapy—this is the minimum time required to awaken the nerve endings and get the draining process underway.

- Before starting your facial therapy, make sure your hair is well back off your face and that you have removed any clothing that might get in the way.

facial therapy

Front shoulders: Place the first two fingers of each hand on your collarbones, at the point where they meet your breastbone. Press the balls of your fingers firmly into the flesh immediately beneath your collarbone and release. Continue this movement as you progress out towards the shoulder joint. This should take about four moves. Return in the same manner to the breastbone. Repeat five times.

Back shoulders: Using the three middle fingers of one hand, massage thoroughly the part of the trapezius muscle located behind the opposite shoulder with small circular movements. Repeat on the other side. Now place your thumb in the hollow behind your collarbones and, using all four fingers, "pinch" all over the muscle repeatedly for as long as you can. Repeat on the other side. Use the same pinching action, with your thumbs pointing downward, on the back of the neck moving up toward the hairline.

Neck: Gently massage your neck from left to right in a rhythmical, upward-stroking motion, with one hand following the other. Continue for two or three minutes. Next, pinch gently all over the front and sides of your neck for a further minute. Finish with two minutes of stroking.

Jawline: Position your thumbs just beneath your chin and the balls of your fingers on top. Now pinch your way along the lower jawbone until you reach the earlobes, applying greater pressure at the corner of the jawbone and just beneath the earlobes. Aim to cover the distance in four pinches and repeat the sequence ten times.

Cheeks: Using the first two fingers of each hand, work along the underside of the cheekbones, pressing the balls of your fingers gently against the bone and then releasing them. Work out toward the point where your cheekbones and upper jawbones meet, then come back toward the center, four or five moves in each direction. Repeat ten times.

Sinus points: Using the balls of your index fingers, apply pressure to the muscles on either side of the nose, starting at the bridge and moving down to the nostrils. Your fingers should be pointing inward so that you feel cartilage rather than bone. Continue for one minute.

Eyes: Close your eyes and feel the bony rims of your eye sockets. Starting at the outer edge, use your third fingers to trace around the rims of the sockets, applying more pressure across your brow and at the point where the eyebrow meets the side of the nose. Do at least ten "laps" at a steady pace, working on both eyes simultaneously.

Forehead: Position your thumbs just above the outer edge of your eyebrows and your index fingers above the inner edge. Pinch in a rhythmical fashion up toward the hairline and back again. Now place your thumbs on your temples and repeat. Continue for a couple of minutes.

Scalp: See Bharti's scalp massage on page 66.

FACT
YOUR FACE IS SWATHED IN MUSCLES. MANY OF THESE
DELICATE, INTERLINKING MUSCLES ARE ATTACHED TO
THE SKIN (AS OPPOSED TO BEING TETHERED TO BONE
AS THEY ARE ELSEWHERE IN THE BODY), WHICH MAKES
THEM VULNERABLE TO DAMAGE FROM HEAVY-HANDED
SKINCARE ROUTINES AND MASSAGE. SO GO GENTLY.

Always be very gentle in your treatment of your neck—this
is because of the delicate nature of the tissue, the underlying
thyroid gland and the proximity of the voice box.

If you are carrying extra weight on your face, regular stimulation
by massage will stop it from looking heavy and bring a glow back
to your cheeks.

Massaging the sides of your nose to clear the sinus points
will help to prevent your sinuses blocking. Once you clear these
points, the area around your eyes will look better and you will
regain your sense of smell.

✳ Avoid lines around the eyes by keeping the skin lightly moisturized, and massage gently to stimulate the lymphatic circulation and thus drain any fluids and toxins that have accumulated. This can also help to prevent dark shadows.

✳ To prevent lines on the forehead, give the flesh a shallow pinch (see facial massage, page 99)—this will also encourage regeneration of the skin.

BALANCE AND INNER HEALTH

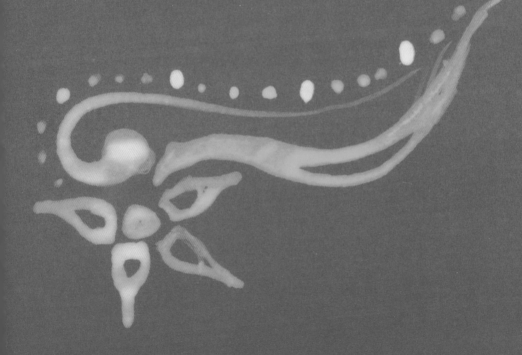

To achieve real radiance, we have to work from the inside as well as the outside, caring for the body and mind internally. Regarding your body as a temple, a place of respect, elevates your experience of life.

Yoga, breathing exercises, and meditation are nonstrenuous and the benefits of spending a few minutes each day practicing them are immense. You can also make a real difference by setting aside quiet time to relax, breathe deeply, and de-stress.

Finally, diet is all-important in promoting health and radiance, so that you will both look and feel great.

RELAXATION

Relaxing is one of the most effective ways of counteracting stress. It diffuses the accumulated physical and psychological pressure so that, when you go back into battle, you feel refreshed and your load feels lighter. This in turn will make you far more able to withstand any stress you do experience, since it will help you to experience it in a more positive way. Stress should also then not invade your life in quite the same way. And stress can be very invasive, affecting our state of mind, our nerves, our posture, and our sleep, as well as our body's ability to carry out its many vital functions effectively.

✻ Take a complete break from time to time, to give your mind and body the opportunity to recharge.

✻ A long, relaxing soak in the bath is one of the most therapeutic treatments you can give yourself (see pages 74–7).

✻ Encourage relaxation habits in your children—play them some soothing music or read them a story during their bath time, so that they come to associate it with relaxation.

BREATHING

Good breathing floods our cells and tissues with dynamic oxygen, which has the power to galvanize cell metabolism and boost cell turnover. The benefits are immediately noticeable in the freshness of our skin tone and the brightness of our eyes. And because everything is running efficiently, we feel more alert and alive. Proper abdominal breathing helps to streamline the midriff and gives your frame underlying strength, discipline, and poise. Steady, deep breathing also cleanses the system by increasing the output of potentially toxic, waste gas and providing some assistance to the lymphatic circulation.

breathing for beauty

Recharge your batteries by concentrating on your breathing for five to ten minutes. Do it either sitting or lying down.

With eyes closed rest your hands on your abdomen and breathe in gently, pushing against your hands as you do so.

Breathe out, lingering over the out-breath until the need for another in-breath naturally arises. Do not exaggerate the inhalation or the exhalation; in fact, the quieter the better.

Continue to observe your breathing until this deeper, slower rhythm has become automatic. Stop when you feel your strength returning.

Good breathing uses the diaphragm, a sheet of muscle between the lungs and ribcage. It is impossible to achieve maximum intake of air if your posture is slumped or tensed.

Rest one hand on your tummy, around your navel, and place the other on your upper chest.

Breathe slowly and deeply and watch where the movement is taking place. When you are breathing well, most of the visible activity appears to be going on in your abdomen, which moves slowly in and out. Breathing should not involve rapid movements of the upper chest. Good breathing can calm and prevent anxious states.

FACT
YAWNING IS THE BODY'S CLEVER WAY OF DELIVERING
A HUGE BLAST OF OXYGEN INTO THE SYSTEM. WE YAWN
WHEN WE ARE TIRED OR WHEN OUR BREATHING BECOMES
SHALLOW DUE TO STRESS OR ANXIETY. MAKE SURE YOU
REALLY LUXURIATE IN THE STRETCH—THIS ALSO HELPS
YOUR MUSCLES TO RELAX.

The warming properties of ginger allow it to liquefy excess mucus, which keeps the passages of the nose and throat clear. It is very effective in clearing the sinuses and even has the potential to reduce asthmatic tendencies.

Respiratory tonic—drink the following every morning on an empty stomach: 6–7 drops freshly squeezed ginger juice (peel a small ginger root, grate it and press it), ½ teaspoon honey in half a glass of hot water.

YOGA

Exercise, in any form, intensifies all the benefits of good breathing. Yoga postures are especially valuable because they teach you to become aware of your breathing and to use it as a means of relaxing, resculpting, and revitalizing your body. When you are in a relaxed state, the oxygen level in your bloodstream is higher and your body is in balance. Proper relaxation also takes the pressure off all body systems and provides an opportunity for much-needed recuperation.

yoga: breathing exercises

Try these breath control exercises that are part of yoga practice. Invigorate your system in the morning with these two routines and you will start the day with a radiant glow.

Close your right nostril with your right thumb and inhale deeply through your left nostril. Close both nostrils and hold the air in your lungs for as long as is comfortable. Next, close your left nostril and exhale slowly through your right nostril. Keep your left nostril closed and inhale through your right nostril. Close both nostrils. Now slowly exhale through your left nostril. This is one cycle or round. Try to do three or four rounds each time.

Now adopt a comfortable sitting position, placing your hands on your knees and lowering your eyes. Inhale and exhale quickly and forcefully, like a pair of bellows. Start with one exhalation per second and gradually increase speed. Aim to complete one cycle of ten exhalations initially and increase gradually.

The second exercise clears the head, the nasal passages and the respiratory system. It brings huge supplies of oxygen into the lungs and draws out large quantities of carbon dioxide from the body, so purifying the blood. It also tones up your heart and activates the respiratory, circulatory, and digestive systems.

DIET

The food you choose becomes you. There is no source of building materials for skin, bones, nerves, and other body tissues other than the food you place in your mouth. If you want a healthy body, eat a healthy diet. A regular intake of the essential vitamins, minerals, fiber, fats, carbohydrates and protein, together with water, is all that it takes to keep the body's complex machinery running smoothly. By supplying our bodies with these nutrients, we are also providing our skin, hair, nails, teeth, muscles and bones with the first-class nourishment that they require. Poor eating habits and digestive problems undermine our general health and increase our susceptibility to illness. In a relatively short time, they can also have a visible impact on our appearance—most noticeably on the condition of our hair, nails, and skin.

Almost as important as the food we take in is the swift and complete disposal of the waste products generated by our consumption. Poor elimination is a serious contributing factor in varicose veins, cellulite, premature lines, and wrinkles, and congested, pimply skin. To combat or prevent constipation, step up your water consumption and intake of dietary fiber with plenty of fresh fruits and vegetables, wholegrains and pulses. This will assist the passage of undigested food through the gut. Other effective antidotes include regular exercise, avoiding refined, processed foods, and building up your abdominal muscles.

Nearly two thirds of our body weight is made up of water. This is stored within the cells, outside the cells and in our body fluids. We need water to aid digestion and elimination. When we don't take in enough, toxins get trapped in our tissues, causing the complexion to deteriorate. Drink eight to ten glasses of water per day.

Excluding wheat and dairy products from your diet for three months will firm up and trim your figure, breathe new life into your skin, and increase your general vitality, by improving your digestion and assimilation of food and keeping your respiratory system clear.

- Eat fruit and vegetables raw whenever possible for their dynamic internal cleansing action and to maximize their food value.

- For a refreshing drink, add a slice of lemon or lime to a glass of cool water. This is an excellent healthy alternative to soft or fizzy drinks.

BHARTI VYAS BALANCE AND INNER HEALTH

how to cook and eat

The way in which you prepare and eat your food can promote health and radiance. Take time to enjoy it!

If you are feeling tense after a stressful day at work, take a few minutes to relax before going into the kitchen.

When you are preparing a meal, place fresh flowers in the kitchen so that you can enjoy the sight and smell as you cook.

Listen to music that calms you as you prepare food.

Handle your food as much as possible—it brings you closer to the ingredients. Enjoy the color, texture, and aromas of the food you cook with.

Keep the kitchen clean and make sure that work surfaces are uncluttered so that you feel organized and calm.

When you eat, chew slowly—taste your food and feel it in your mouth.

Eat at a table—slouching distorts the digestive system, promoting indigestion.

Even for a simple meal, place flowers on the table and use candles at night.

❧ Include a salad in most meals. Remember: any raw vegetables (or fruit) can be incorporated; there's no need to stick to tried-and-tested combinations.

❧ Eat plenty of iron-rich spinach, watercress, and parsley to keep up your hemoglobin level, particularly just before a period and during pregnancy.

❧ Dark green vegetables are a good source of calcium for nails, teeth, and bones.

※ Millet is a useful food for promoting healthy, lustrous hair. It contains seven of the eight amino acids your hair needs. Stir millet flakes into muesli or use it instead of rice and pasta.

※ Poultry and game contain less fat than other meats, plus the important B vitamins and iron. Avoid processed meats.

※ Fish is a great and healthy source of protein. Eat at least two portions a week. Essential fatty acids in oily fish and shellfish help to keep skin moist and strengthen hair and nails.

Pumpkin, sesame, and sunflower seeds are nutritional treasure troves packed with protein, fiber, and many skin-saving and beautifying nutrients.

Combine nuts and seeds, pulses and wholegrains for a highly nutritious cocktail of plant-based proteins, e.g. peanut butter on toast, hummus and pittas. Pulses are an excellent low-fat, high-fiber source of protein.

Make sure all the oils you buy are cold-pressed and unrefined—that is, nutritionally intact. Fry only with olive and sesame oil, as these remain "stable" at high temperatures, but never heat to smoking point. Corn and sunflower oil can be used for gentle frying.

To preserve your eyes and your eyesight, eat plenty of fruit and vegetables, poultry, fish, nuts, wholegrains, seeds and their oils. Opt for orange-colored fruits and vegetables, dark green, leafy vegetables, and avocados whenever possible.

BHARTI VYAS BALANCE AND INNER HEALTH

- Zinc helps to fight infection and aids the process of wound healing. Good sources include wholegrain cereals, egg yolk, dairy products, and red meat.

- Zinc works with vitamin C so plan your meals to include fresh vegetables and fruits along with zinc-rich foods.

- Zinc and copper work together to slow the deterioration of your skin—life-bearing foods (nuts, grains, and pulses) are good sources of both mineral micronutrients.

🌿 If you are dairy-intolerant but concerned about your calcium intake, other good sources of calcium are tinned sardines and pilchards, parsley, leafy green vegetables such as broccoli, spinach and watercress, dried figs, soya flour, almonds, sesame seeds, Indian tea, curry powder, dry mustard, canned salmon and eggs.

🌿 If you find your digestion improves after eliminating cows' milk products from your diet, but you would like to enjoy some form of cheese or milk, try products made from ewes', goats,' or buffalo milk.

Tofu, apricots, and prunes are good sources of calcium. Enjoy these in your diet for strong bones and healthy muscles.

Coarse hair, dry skin and lethargy may be signs of low iodine levels in the diet. Good sources of iodine include iodized salt, seafood, and seaweed.

your food allies

Apricots: Apricots are a rich source of beta-carotene, folic acid, and iron.

Avocado pears: Rich in potassium and the vital antioxidant triad of vitamins A, C, and E, avocados also contain easily digested monounsaturated fats. The pulp is thought to contain antifungal and antibacterial compounds, and substances that stimulate collagen development in skin, thus increasing its elasticity.

Asafoetida: Don't let its smell put you off! It subdues wind and nasal mucus, aids gastric processes, strengthens the heart and regulates the menstrual cycle. It can also be used in the treatment of rheumatism, deafness, paralysis, and eye disease.

Aubergines: Aubergine contains plant compounds that are thought to prevent cancer and act as powerful antioxidants.

Cabbage: A rich source of iron, cabbage is thought to help prevent certain cancers.

Cardamom: Chew cardamom pods to sweeten the breath—this also stimulates digestion, relieves the symptoms of indigestion, and can help calm vomiting.

Cinnamon: Cinnamon helps decongest the nasal passages, and helps prevent flatulence, diarrhea, and indigestion. It's a good tonic for your system at the start of the day.

Crucifers: Scientific evidence shows that green plants of the Crucifer family contain powerful anti-cancer substances. Enjoy at least one portion of the following each day: broccoli, cauliflower, cabbage, kale, Brussels sprouts, turnips, mustard greens, and kohlrabi.

Cumin: Cumin seeds relieve colic and indigestion.

Dates: Dates are a good source of minerals needed for good health, and aid the digestive system by acting as a mild laxative.

Fresh coriander (cilantro): The most widely used herb in the world, it is said to reduce stomach upset.

Garlic: Garlic contains natural antifungal, antibacterial, and antiviral compounds. Research suggests that garlic helps reduce blood cholesterol levels, lower blood pressure, and prevent abnormal blood clots

Ginger: Added to food, or eaten alone, root ginger aids digestion and is effective against many forms of motion sickness and nausea.

Lentils: Lentils contain good quantities of B-complex vitamins, iron and protein. To enhance the absorption of iron from lentils, be sure to include a food rich in vitamin C, such as peppers, at the same meal.

Melons: These fruits stimulate the kidneys, and aid in a cleansing diet.

Milk and dairy products: These are good sources of protein, calcium and B-complex vitamins. However, dairy foods are not easy for everyone to digest—if you suffer from dairy-intolerance, try products made from ewes', goats,' or buffalo milk. The range of non-cows' milk products has increased hugely over the past few years.

Mustard: Mustard seeds are an ancient remedy for headache and flu.

Onions: Compounds in onions are thought to reduce blood cholesterol levels, lower blood pressure, and prevent blood clots. There is strong evidence that they are also rich in natural antibiotics.

Soya (soy) beans: As well as providing good-quality protein and host of nutrient compounds, recent medical research suggests the oestrogen-like substances in soya beans can reduce the unpleasant side effects of menopause, and may help protect against breast cancer.

Tamarind: Tamarind is rich in vitamins and is said to be a tonic for the kidneys and liver.

Turmeric: Turmeric has been used for centuries as a liver tonic and to relieve digestive problems.

Walnuts: These nuts are a vital source of fats (omega-3 fatty acids) that help maintain a healthy heart, boost the immune system, and protect joints from certain forms of arthritis.

SLEEP

Sleep is a wonderfully inexpensive pleasure as well as being a very important part of the body's repair mechanism. It is the time when your body repairs tissue cells and when your mind sifts and sorts the subconscious superfluities of the day. Without enough sleep we are more prone to depression and less able to concentrate and make the right decisions about life.

If you want a good night's sleep, avoid eating protein-rich foods after 6 PM: they take much longer to digest. Try to eat your evening meal before 7 PM.

If you're having trouble sleeping, try to go to bed at the same time each night and extend the ritual into a bedtime routine that will set the mood for sleep.

If you can't sleep, check your room isn't too hot: a temperature of 64–75 degrees is perfect for uninterrupted sleep.

Spend around 20 minutes in a lukewarm bath before you go to bed: light a candle, play some music, and burn some incense. Go to bed immediately after you've dried yourself and had a glass of cool water.

If you wake up in the night with your head running full of lists and worries, get up and go into another room to make a list of the issues on your mind. Sleep is likely to come much more easily once you return to your atmosphere of restful slumber.

Sleeping habits can compound posture-related problems. Reduce your pillow heights if you feel any strain in your neck. The purpose of a pillow is to fill the gap between your ear and your shoulder while keeping your head at a right angle to your neck.

WELL-BEING

To maintain your general health and well-being, it is important to try to minimize the amount of stress in your life. Although you may have no control over external factors, there are many easy ways in which you can reduce and deal with the effects of stress on your body and mind (see also Relaxation, Yoga, and Breathing).

stress-busting exercise

Sit back in your chair.

Hang your arms by your sides, pulling your shoulders down and back.

Take a deep breath, expanding your chest and filling your lungs to capacity.

Breathe in and out very deeply, concentrating on the rise and fall of your abdomen.

Do this five times, then breathe normally, counting to three as you inhale and four as you exhale.

If you suffer from anxiety attacks, take a hot bath, adding two heaped tablespoons of ginger and the same amount of baking soda to the water. Shut your eyes and breathe in the vapors.

A quick fix to soothe a racing heart beat is a cup of orange juice with a pinch of ground nutmeg and a teaspoon of honey.

A headache may be telling you to enjoy a drink of water or juice. At these times, avoid tea and coffee. The caffeine they contain acts as a mild diuretic and encourages the body to flush out more fluids.

emergency weekend treatment

Make one weekend a month a mini-cleansing celebration. Return to work on Monday a calmer, refreshed, more uplifted soul. Your friends and colleagues will instantly notice your new radiance!

Drink boiled water with herbs infused in it instead of stimulants such as tea and coffee. Add peppermint or coriander, or at the very least use shop-bought tisanes.

Avoid alcohol, cigarettes, and processed food.

Wear loose, comfortable, light clothes.

Think invigorating walks rather than extreme exercise.

Splash out on organic vegetables and fruit; eat simply but well.

Turn off the television, and seek your stimulation from reading, conversation, painting, or quiet contemplation.

Make sure you sleep for at least nine hours a night.

Have frequent warm baths.

Pamper yourself with candles, aromatherapy oils, incense, and soothing music.

Treat yourself to a divine bath of the five nectars:

In Ayurveda, milk, honey, yogurt, ghee, and banana are considered to be the five perfect foods. Combine the mashed pulp of a banana with two tablespoons of milk, one teaspoonful of honey, one teaspoon of yogurt, and one of ghee. Massage the sweet-scented mix onto your skin and plunge into a warm bath to nourish, soften, smooth, and re-energize your skin.

COMMON PROBLEMS

Unfortunately, most people suffer from problems with their appearance or general health at some point. If you deal with the problem quickly and effectively, it need never become an issue in your life. Many common ailments can be treated without resorting to expensive lotions and potions. In this section, I have recommended lots of home treatments and exercises to help with a variety of complaints.

SCALP

Scalp problems are extremely common, ranging from oily and dry scalps, scaliness, itchiness, smelly scalps, to tight scalps, and sponginess. The most effective way to keep your scalp in good working order is to massage it regularly with oil. The physical impact of regular massage on your scalp is to keep the maximum number of follicles active and increase the strength and diameter of each hair. The movements of your hands and fingers act on the blood vessels beneath the surface and on the follicles themselves. Manipulating your scalp also helps to release tension, which improves the general flow of blood and rectifies any underlying imbalances. As an extra bonus, during a massage the natural scalp oils are smoothed along the length of the hair.

If you are suffering from any of the scalp problems mentioned here, try Bharti's special Scalp Massage (see page 66).

HAIR

Hair problems can be highly upsetting for sufferers, since our hair is an immediate and highly visible indication of our age and general health. In many cases, hair lacks condition and health simply due to overtreating it—if the hair is stripped of its natural protective coating of oil, the inside of the hair shaft is vulnerable to damage and moisture evaporation, which results in weakened hair and split ends. A healthy balanced diet will help the general health of your hair, as will regular scalp massages (see page 66).

Hair loss and thinning hair, including male baldness, is generally caused by hormonal disruption—natural or induced—or hereditary factors beyond our control. High stress levels result in constricted circulation to the scalp, which is equivalent to cutting off the hair's food and water supply. Regular massage can help to make the most of the hair you have by boosting growth and conditioning hair to give the impression of bulk. If massage becomes a way of life at an early age, it is possible to inhibit an inherited tendency.

Graying occurs when insufficient melanin pigment is produced in the hair follicle to maintain our original hair color. It is also sometimes linked to an iron deficiency. Many of us choose to color our hair because we do not feel or want to look the age our changing hair color suggests. Provided you take the trouble to protect and condition your hair and scalp, there's no reason why you shouldn't dye your hair.

To give an impresson of volume in fine hair or camouflaging in graying hair, try highlights or lowlights—highlights give the hair a sun-dappled appearance, while lowlights introduce deeper glints.

If you are trying to disguise gray hair, don't use henna—it tinges the gray hairs bright red and therefore identifies the very hairs you are attempting to disguise.

Vegetable dyes provide the most natural cover for gray hair, and the best effect is obtained with a dye a shade lighter than your own.

When dyeing your own hair, always wear gloves and apply a smear of moisturizing cream around the hairline to protect the skin.

If your hair is looking limp and dull, oil the hair with coconut oil—comb a small amount through your hair, from roots to ends, and leave overnight for a glossy head of hair.

Cider vinegar (for dark hair and flaky/dandruff scalps) or lemon juice (for fair hair and greasy scalps) added to a basin of water as a final rinse will restore sheen and maintain the acid balance of your hair.

※ To treat dandruff, mix one egg yolk with a squirt of lime juice and a few drops of camphor and apply to your scalp for ten minutes. This will reintroduce missing protein to your scalp. Rinse with warm water.

※ Hair loss tends to happen at times of physical and emotional stress—diet is a key factor in preventing thinning. Stick to healthy foods and increase your intake of fruit and vegetables to give your hair follicles the nutrients they need.

PIMPLES

Pimples are a real pain, whatever age you are.
Blemishes and acne develop when the sebum "plug"
that blocks the hair follicle becomes infected by
bacteria that usually live harmlessly on the skin,
causing the sebaceous glands to become inflamed.
Attempts to de-grease the skin with harsh
cleansers and toners often aggravate the problem
by stimulating sebaceous activity and so further
disturbing the skin's protective covering.

If you suffer from recurrent acne, you will probably have been told by your doctor whether it is caused by a hormonal imbalance and may have been prescribed medication. While it is essential to work with your doctor to prevent any infection, you should be aware that any medication you do take will have some side-effect within the body, such as the disturbance of the friendly bacteria in the intestines by antibiotics, for example. Your own habits can help to reduce the severity of attacks and the likelihood of cross-infection (see overleaf).

FACT
**PIMPLY FOREHEAD: CONSTIPATION AND A CLOGGED
LYMPHATIC SYSTEM ARE OFTEN AT THE ROOT OF THE
PROBLEM—THE SKIN IS THE BODY'S MAIN ORGAN OF
ELIMINATION AND WHEN THE WASTE IS NOT DISPOSED
OF ANY OTHER WAY, IT MAY BE EXCRETED VIA THE SKIN.**

- If you have an outbreak of pimples on your forehead, avoid touching them—the oils from your fingers simply "nourish" the pimples as well as carrying bacteria to the area.

- To avoid pimples, try cutting back on your consumption of sugar, refined carbohydrates, and saturated fats. A gentle detox program, excluding wheat and dairy products from your diet, will reduce the potential irritants in the blood and calm the activities of the sebaceous glands.

blackheads

If you suffer from excess blackheads, try these home remedies:

Add half a teaspoon of Epsom salts to a cup of warm water, and wash your face by dipping a cotton ball into the liquid.

Grind up fresh parsley into a pulp and apply to the oily area prone to blackheads, lie down for 15 minutes to encourage blood circulation to the face, then cleanse, nourish, and moisturize as normal.

❧ Use a spot treatment with anti-bacterial and antiseptic properties, such as a camphor-based preparation, to help control inflammation and cross-infection.

❧ Wash pimply skin two or three times each day with a cleansing bar or soap-free facial wash to remove skin "grease" and control the spread of bacteria.

❧ Moisturize pimply skin with an oil-free formulation.

❧ Always remove all your make-up before going to bed. Any products remaining on your face will block your pores, causing pimples.

FACT
HORMONAL FLUCTUATIONS DISTURB THE ACTIVITIES OF
OUR SEBACEOUS GLANDS, RESULTING IN OVERACTIVITY
AND BLOCKAGES, LEADING TO BLACKHEADS, OPEN PORES
AND PIMPLES. THIS EXPLAINS WHY WE SOMETIMES GET
PIMPLES ON OUR CHIN JUST BEFORE A PERIOD.

- Do not try to exfoliate pimply skin—this stimulates the sebaceous glands in the dermis to produce more oil.

- To keep the skin around the jawline clear of blemishes, pinch and drain the jawline in the direction of your earlobe, where there is a lymph gland waiting to filter out toxins—do this exercise two or three times a day until the skin is improved, then once a week to keep skin clear.

- Apply a turmeric and honey healing mask (see page 85) directly to pimples.

🌿 Avoid touching and picking pimples because of the risk of
scarring and pigmentation marks.

🌿 If you suffer from acne in your teenage years, very gently
stimulate the area around each spot with your fingers.
The infection will be brought into the shaft of the pimple and
it will encourage blood flow into the damaged follicle,
healing it faster.

🌿 Mid-life acne is caused by changing hormone levels—
try to drink more water to flush out the facial tissues, and
make sure you eat more fresh fruit, vegetables, and salad,
wholegrains, live yogurt, seeds and nuts and fresh fish.

If you do have an outbreak of mid-life acne, cleanse and moisturize with almond oil softened in the palm of your hand. Massage your skin delicately with a gentle "palming" action to calm your irritated nerve endings.

To calm acne-ridden, sensitive skin, make a healing face mask by mixing almond powder (grind almonds in a blender) with a few teaspoons of water, apply to your face and let dry for half an hour before rinsing.

WRINKLES

Most people develop wrinkles as they grow older, due to falling moisture levels and dwindling supplies of elastin (elastin links with the collagen fibers in the skin and they lose their ability to stretch). In addition, reduced blood flow deprives the cells of vital nutrients and encourages waste build-up at a stage of life when cell reproduction and turnover are already on the wane. This deterioration and degeneration sounds alarming, but it occurs gradually over the space of several decades, at a pace broadly determined by your genes. However, it can be hastened or arrested by a number of factors, including sun damage, smoking, poor diet, stress, lifestyle abuse, and misguided skincare or skin neglect, which are in your power to influence. No-one can delay this process indefinitely, but your skin does not have to show your age if you adopt a healthy skincare routine and look after your general health.

Drinking plenty of water and eating nutrient-rich food will nourish your body's tissues and help waste toxins to pass through, rather than accumulate. If your circulation is poor, you will be able to read this in your skin. Your skin will gradually become thinner, less elastic and fine lines will appear, leading to full-blown crags and wrinkles. There are three key elements to avoiding the so-called "inevitable" ravages of age: eating healthily, flushing the system with lots of water, and polishing/massaging the surface of the skin. Regular facial massages can help (see page 96).

Wrinkles also point to a drop in the skin's oil and moisture (water is required to keep the collagen fibers in your skin pliable). Boosting your vitamin C intake can also help.

❀ Wrinkles on the forehead: be aware of when you are wrinkling your forehead or furrowing your brow and consciously relax the muscles to smooth out the skin.

❀ To avoid premature lines on the forehead, use a mild, oil-based cleanser or almond oil to avoid stripping the skin of its natural oil and moisture. Remove cleanser with a damp facial sponge.

❀ Tone with cold water or rosewater—avoid astringent preparations as they can aggravate the skin.

OTHER SKIN PROBLEMS...

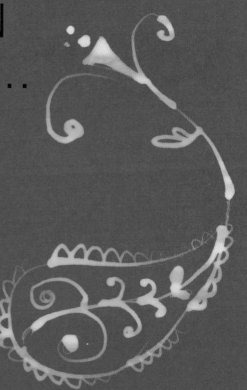

COLD SORES

Apply aloe vera gel to cold-sore blisters, or if you are feeling adventurous, buy some bitter ghee from an Indian supermarket and use it like an ointment several times a day.

ECZEMA

If you suffer from sporadic outbreaks of eczema, do some detective work to try to find the trigger. Watch your diet, being particularly aware of reactions to common food allergens such as wheat and dairy products, citrus fruits, spices, and alcohol.

DRY CHEEKS

If the skin on your cheeks is prone to dryness, use a gentle, cream-based cleanser and wash it off with a damp natural sponge or cotton wool pad.

The Nourishing Cheek Face Mask (see page 88) will help loosen dead cells on dry cheeks, enabling healthy new ones to take their place.

PSORIASIS

Psoriasis is caused by internal problems that accelerate the cell division, and unfortunately the skin shreds off very slowly, leaving scaly patches—after bathing, apply ghee to the affected area, and take daily supplements of primrose oil, vitamin E, and cod-liver oil, which encourage the skin to lubricate.

IRREGULAR PIGMENTATION

This problem can occur on all areas of the body. Uneven pigmentation or mottling can be caused by fluctuating female hormones, food allergens floating in the bloodstream, and exposure to the sun, not to mention a rough-and-ready approach to skincare!

FACT
SOME WOMEN ARE PRONE TO DEVELOP DARKER PATCHES OF SKIN
ON THE FACE AS A RESULT OF THE HORMONAL CHANGES THAT TAKE
PLACE DURING PREGNANCY, MENOPAUSE, AND WHILE TAKING THE
CONTRACEPTIVE PILL. HORMONALLY RELATED PIGMENTATION SHOULD
CORRECT ITSELF, BUT IF THE PATCHES DO NOT DISAPPEAR WITHIN
SIX MONTHS, SEE YOUR DOCTOR TO CHECK HORMONE LEVELS.

If you suffer from irregular pigmentation, keep your skincare routine as simple as possible—avoid harsh sponges, cleanse with pH-balanced soap and water, and don't use toner.

To improve a mottled skin tone, use a heavy moisturizer, ideally with built-in UV sunscreen. Alternatively apply a fine sunscreen to the face after moisturizing—SPF 15 is recommended year-round by dermatologists.

Avoid skincare products containing oil of bergamot, as this accelerates the tanning process.

If you notice pigmentation marks developing on your cheeks, start wearing a high-protection sunscreen at all times.

- A vitamin B–complex supplement, supported by a balanced diet, may help to clear liver spots.

- If you have small marks or areas of discoloration on the chin and jawline, apply a mild cleansing lotion or almond oil to the area and massage gently using the balls of the first two fingers, paying particular attention to the indentation just above your chin.

- To avoid rings of lighter skin around the neck, always hold yourself as tall and straight as you can and extend your neck to its maximum length.

- To disperse melanin build-up, exfoliate your neck once a week with the All-purpose Oatmeal Scrub (see page 84), using the minimum finger pressure.

EXCESS HAIR...

Excess facial and body hair can be very upsetting and confidence-shattering for women and girls, but try not to despair. Excess hair is quite common: 25 percent of women have noticeable hair on their face. The reason for this is the male hormone testosterone, but its influence is normally obscured by estrogen—this is why at the time of the menopause when estrogen levels begin to fall, facial hair often increases.

You can try using depilatory creams, plucking, waxing, or epilation, but be aware that creams can irritate sensitive skin. The only sure way to remove facial hair permanently is by laser treatment, but always discuss the options with your beauty consultant before embarking on a course of treatment (see the advice on pages 178–80).

DOWNY HAIR ON FOREHEAD

If you notice that your children have downy hair on the upper part of the forehead, rub gently with a towel after a bath— this helps to wear out the fine hairs without stimulating the follicle to become stronger.

If you have visible downy hair on your forehead, rub a freshly cut lemon gently over the hair—leave for five to seven minutes before rinsing off. Repeat whenever the darker new growth appears.

❧ Cleanse areas of downy hair gently with pH-balanced soap and water so as not to overstimulate the area.

❧ Use water-based moisturizer on patches of downy hair to give as little nourishment as possible to the hairs.

HAIR ON CHEEKS

✽ If a child has a tendency to facial hair, encourage gentle rubbing with a face cloth as part of the morning wash or bathtime routine.

✽ If facial hair is a problem, follow a skincare routine that does not irritate or stimulate your skin—use a Lemon-based mask (see page 87) and repeat once a month, or when darker regrowth appears.

✽ To avoid stimulating facial hair, tone with rosewater (this has a calming effect), use a very light moisturizer and cleanse gently with pH-balanced soap and water.

HAIR ON UPPER LIP

Hair removing and bleaching creams on the upper lip can damage the tissue and sometimes cause premature lines and wrinkles—always do a patch test on the skin first, and if you feel an itching sensation or your skin becomes inflamed after application, remove the cream immediately and do not attempt to use it again.

To prevent the build-up of facial hair, from an early age rub the affected skin gently with a towel/face cloth or bleach with lemon juice.

TREATMENTS FOR UNWANTED HAIR

For many years, electrolysis was thought to be the most effective treatment for hair removal, but its side effects involved degeneration of skin cells, and sometimes permanent marking or scarring. Recent research has found the use of lasers and light therapy to be a highly effective and safe route to permanent hair removal.

Note: Consult a reputable therapist before embarking on any salon treatment for unwanted hair.

INTENSE PULSE LIGHT (IPL)

Intense Pulse Light (IPL) removes hair by pulsating heat through the skin, but because it works on variable light wavelengths rather than a fixed beam, it is more comfortable for the recipient. Although your skin will probably be a bit swollen and pink afterwards, it should quickly heal without scarring.

LASERS

There are various laser sources in use, including Ruby lasers, Alexandrite lasers, Nd:YAG lasers, and Diode lasers, some of which are more suitable for certain types of skin than others. Your therapist will advise you on this if you decide to undergo a course of treatment. Lasers can treat small areas like the upper lip, as well as larger areas like the back or legs. The Nd: YAG laser can directly target the melanin in the hair structure and not the melanin in the skin, which makes it effective in treating darker skins.

IPL and laser treatment are expensive but worth the investment, as not only do they work in permanently removing unwanted hair, but they stop the dehydration of the skin cells.

FACT
LACK OF SLEEP AND SENSITIVITY TO CERTAIN SKIN AND
MAKE-UP PRODUCTS ARE THE MOST COMMON CAUSES OF
PUFFY EYES—SLUGGISH CIRCULATION CAN SOMETIMES
PLAY A PART. PUFFY EYES MAY ALSO INDICATE A THYROID
PROBLEM OR SIGNAL CONSTIPATION.

PUFFY EYES

It is said that the eyes are the windows to the
soul, and they are also an immediate indication
of our tiredness and state of health.

 To soothe puffy eyes, soak black tea bags in warm water
(or, if you prefer, cotton balls dipped in witch hazel) and
place upon your closed eyes for 15 minutes.

BHARTI VYAS COMMON PROBLEMS

DARK CIRCLES

Dark circles under the eyes can be brought on by a shortage of sleep, poor circulation, or poor elimination. Dark circles also occur as a result of kidney problems, food intolerance, or various nutritional deficiencies.

The problem of dark circles can soon become deep-seated unless it is properly addressed. Make sure you drink at least 8 glasses of water a day to encourage the elimination of toxins from the body.

TIRED EYES

To brighten up tired eyes, catch up on lost hours of sleep with a few early nights (bringing your bedtime forward by an hour or more pays dividends).

Relieve and rest tired eyes by placing cotton wool pads soaked in water over your eyes—it will reduce the blood flow to the area and help to remove toxic build-up in the eye muscles and tissue.

Rest your eyes regularly when you are reading, writing, or using a computer monitor (ideally, take a 10-minute break every couple of hours).

Droopy eyes are caused by a lack of muscle tone in the upper eyelid, combined with the downward force of gravity. If massaged regularly over a period of time, it is possible to regain some degree of tone.

CROWS' FEET

Crows' feet are natural lines of expression—if the skin around the eyes is well-moisturized they add to the character of the face. Only if the skin is allowed to become dry do they become deeply etched.

Lightly moisturize the delicate skin beside the eyes with almond oil, but don't pull or rub the skin—smooth in gently with the fingertips.

EYEBROWS

If you are sensitive to pain and find plucking your eyebrows difficult, gently pull upward on the outside edge of your eyebrow while you pluck. Tolerance of pain also appears to be reduced during menstruation, so delay your reshaping until mid-cycle if your pain threshold is low.

MOUTH

The health of your lips and mouth is often indicative of your general lifestyle and diet. The tongue, in particular, is an indicator of vitamin and mineral deficiencies and bad diet.

As well as eating healthily and drinking plenty of water, improve your oral hygiene routine, thoroughly brushing teeth at least twice a day and flossing regularly.

LIPS

If you want to avoid pucker lines and wrinkles on the upper lip, don't smoke—it can add years to your face, as can a tendency to pout. Sun damage is another major culprit.

DEHYDRATED/CRACKED LIPS

Cracking of the skin on the lips is caused by dehydration—resist the desire to lick dry lips for temporary relief as this only makes them dryer still.

Use lip balm as a protection for dry lips—apply several times a day.

FURRY TONGUE

If your tongue is furry, rub it with a small, freshly sliced piece of ginger. This also works for general fungal infections in the mouth.

DOUBLE CHIN

A double chin is usually a sign of weight gain, although the jawline can also become inflated with fluid and toxins due to sluggish lymphatic circulation. Correct posture can also help to avoid a double chin, so pay attention to the way you hold your head—it should just be evenly balanced on the neck column.

To avoid a double chin, watch your food intake and keep up your water consumption, as this will help to sluice out trapped toxins.

double trouble

To tone up a double chin, repeat the following exercise several times daily:

Position your thumbs beneath your chin, your three middle fingers of both hands on top, and pinch.

Resume your position, press firmly, and glide your fingers a little way along your jawline.

Pinch again and repeat the procedure until you reach the corners of your jawbone. Apply sustained pressure here for a few seconds and just beneath your earlobes.

You should see a dramatic improvement within three months.

LOOSE SKIN ON NECK

Do not wait until you see tell-tale rings and crêpiness appearing on your neck before learning the benefits of protecting this fragile skin from dehydration and environmental damage.

❀ To treat loose skin around the neck, gently stimulate the area using the palms of your hands in a sweeping action, and nourish the skin with almond oil. Repeat night and morning.

❀ If the skin on the neck has become crêpey, exfoliate daily with the All-purpose Oatmeal Scrub (see page 84) for an initial period of three weeks, then reducing to once a week. Apply almond oil as a nourishing moisturizer.

❀ If you have a problem with fat build-up on your neck, apply a light film of almond oil all over the neck and, using all four fingers, "pinch" the front, sides, and back for a few minutes. Continue daily for a period of three months.

neck exercises

To strengthen and firm neck muscles:

Keeping your chin level, turn your head to one side so that the chin is over your shoulder. Incline the head backward in a "come hither" movement. Repeat on the other side. Repeat the sequence five times.

Hold your head in a central position, then lean it as far over as you can toward one shoulder and hold for a count of 10. Your neck may feel stiff to begin with. Repeat on the other side, making sure that your shoulders remain still and relaxed throughout. Do five repetitions.

ARMS

Sluggish circulation and build-up of toxins can cause flabby, flaccid arms. Make sure you work your arm muscles and massage to discourage accumulation of toxins and fluids.

WEAK AND TIRED ARM MUSCLES

If the muscles in your arms feel weak and tired, rub olive or almond oil into the skin of your forearm using upward strokes after your bath or before you go to bed. Continue for three minutes.

HANDS

Our hands bear the brunt of extreme weather conditions and cannot escape constant contact with water and detergents, so are extremely vulnerable. Over time, repeated exposure to water and the elements without adequate protection can result in dehydration and discoloration of the skin—in other words, prematurely aged hands. Never stint on the hand cream, even if you think your hands are still in their prime.

aching hands

Prolonged contact with water is not usually recommended for the hands. However, a soak in salt water can soothe aches and pains if undertaken on a regular basis. Always moisturize with hand cream after treatment.

If you have stiff, aching hands or any swelling or puffiness, soak your hands in salt water for 15–20 minutes every day for a two-week period. The most effortless way to do this is while in the bath. Rinse with fresh water and push back the cuticles with a damp flannel.

NAILS

If you look after your hands, you can also preserve
the health and beauty of your nails. Nail problems
(soft or brittle nails, splitting nails, ridges, and white
spots, etc.) are often caused by dietary deficiencies,
so take care of your vitamin and protein intake.

- If you have a tendency to flaky, chipped, dehydrated, or thickened nails, file the free edges of the nails daily and apply a nail strengthener every night to hold the cell layer together.

- White flecks in nails are a sign of an injury or zinc deficiency. Eggs, lentils, and chickpeas are good sources of zinc.

- If the cuticles start to overhang the nail or become dehydrated, ease them back gently using a flannel when they are nicely softened after a soak in the bath. Alternatively use a cotton wool bud after applying cream or oil.

FEET

You may never have beautiful feet—very few people do—but you will certainly have healthy, respectable feet if you soak your feet regularly in a salt bath (see page 76), exfoliate, and use foot cream or almond oil.

FACT
HARD SKIN AND CALLUSES ARE CAUSED BY INAPPROPRIATE
FOOTWEAR, THE EFFECT OF POOR POSTURE AND GENERAL
WEAR AND TEAR ON THE FEET. THEY CAN BECOME VERY
THICK AND LEATHERY IF THE UNDERLYING CAUSE IS NOT
ADDRESSED AND THE FEET NOT PROPERLY CARED FOR.

If you have athlete's foot, swab the affected area with tea tree oil, a natural antiseptic. Then mix one teaspoon of aloe vera gel with a large pinch of turmeric and apply to the itchy parts of your feet before you go to bed. Do this for two weeks.

Cool burning feet with sandalwood oil or mango juice.

To remove hard skin on top of bony areas, rub with a pumice stone or an abrasive scrub after soaking.

FAT AND CELLULITE

Many of us will never have a washboard stomach, and in fact, there is something very feminine about a slightly rounded tummy and curving hips—most of us feel that a less angular silhouette is a fair trade-off for a life lived to the fullest. We should, however, guard against the progressive loss of muscle tone, which has implications for health as well as our figures. Moreover, accumulation of fat encourages wastes and fluid to accumulate, often resulting in cellulite, which is both unhealthy and unsightly.

FLABBY TUMMY

✿ To tone up a flabby tum, activate the flesh on your abdomen using brisk pinching movements. Do it after your bath, having first lubricated the skin with body lotion or oil.

✿ For stretch marks, increase your intake of vitamin E in food or supplement form during vulnerable periods. You could also pierce a vitamin E capsule, squeeze out its contents and rub into the skin of the abdomen.

FLABBY BUTTOCKS

Exfoliate your buttocks at bath times using a mildly abrasive mitt, lubricated with a squirt of bath gel. This will remove dead cells and help to even out the skin's pigments. Moisturize well afterwards.

Massage body lotion into your buttocks using small pinching movements. This activates nerve endings in the skin, which enhances muscle tone and aids detoxification.

CELLULITE

Deposits of cellulite are actually reserves of liquid waste that the body is unable to expel by normal means. It is caused mainly by leading an unhealthy lifestyle. Brisk walking, rebounding (boucing on a mini-trampoline), swimming, and cycling are highly recommended for toning the big leg muscles. Rebounding is a great weapon in the battle against cellulite.

To avoid cellulite build-up, eat plenty of fresh fruit and vegetables (organic when possible), wholegrains, pulses, fish, and chicken. Drink 8–10 glasses of water daily, and cut back on your consumption of coffee, tea, fat, sugar, salt, and alcohol.

Dry skin brushing with a natural bristle brush on your thighs before your bath or shower boosts peripheral circulation and aids the flow of lymph while exfoliating the skin. Always brush in the direction of the heart and avoid broken or sore areas of skin.

VARICOSE VEINS

Varicose veins are usually an inherited condition but you can delay and minimize their appearance (see overleaf).

to prevent or relieve varicose veins

Put your feet up at the end of the day to assist the return of blood to the heart. The feet need to be raised above the level of the head for at least 15–20 minutes to be really effective. Brisk walking to contract leg muscles will also help to push the blood in the right direction.

Wear support tights when you are going to be standing for long periods.

Train yourself out of crossing your legs as this impedes the circulation.

Take a daily supplement of vitamin E.

Reduce your consumption of refined, sugary foods and step up your intake of grains and fresh fruit and vegetables. Citrus fruits, apricots, grapes, blackberries, cherries, broccoli, avocados, nuts, seed oils, and buckwheat all help to strengthen and improve the elasticity of blood vessels.

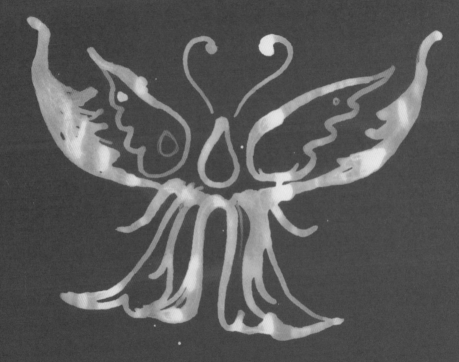

MAKE-UP

Make-up is an essential beauty tool for many women, and there is no reason why you shouldn't use it to enhance your best features—as long as it is applied properly and subtly. It can also act like a magic wand, although in the long run you should be looking to your diet and general health if skin problems don't clear up quickly. Most of us can't afford our own make-up artist, but there are some make-up basics you can learn.

SOLVING PROBLEMS

Although make-up can conceal imperfections, it can also cause them if not applied properly or cleaned off thoroughly, or if you are using the wrong type of make-up for your skin type. Always treat your skin with respect, and if possible, use the best-quality make-up you can afford.

🌸 Always remove your make-up before going to bed—
   the oils in it clog up the pores and make breakouts more likely.

🌸 A layer of moisturizer creates a good base for and a barrier
   against make-up. Leave for 10 minutes and tissue off excess
   before applying foundation.

🌸 If you have lines on your forehead, use an oil-based
   foundation, applied with a damp sponge, then set with
   translucent loose powder.

🌸 If you are prone to pimples, use an oil-free, non-comedogenic
   foundation, such as a silicone-based product. Dab foundation
   on top of pimples, then follow with a light overall application.

Camouflage pimples with concealer after applying foundation, then dust with the finest covering of translucent powder.

If you suffer from irregular pigmentation of your skin, try to wear foundation a shade slightly darker than the pigmented area—apply all over the face, including ears, eyes, and neck, to give uniform tone. Set with translucent loose powder.

Avoid using foundation in areas where you have downy hair (usually around the forehead) as it may highlight the hairs.

For a natural look or if you suffer from excess facial hair, try a tinted moisturizer instead of foundation.

Use a creamy concealer to camouflage dark circles and shadows around the eyes and pat gently with the pad of your middle finger to blend. Finish with a fine application of translucent powder.

If your eyebrows or eyelashes are too fair for your liking, have them tinted a darker shade—eyelashes also look more glossy and striking when they have been tinted. Always have it done professionally—it is safer and the effect is longer-lasting.

Consider semi-permanent make-up, especially if your eyebrows have been overplucked, or you need to camouflage any birth marks or scar tissue, or even if failing eyesight means applying make-up is difficult for you.

✳ To make thin lips look fuller, wear pale colors and add a dab of gloss to the middle of the lips (this makes all lips appear more voluptuous).

✳ If your lips are fuller than you'd like, stick to deeper tones and avoid screamingly bright colors and too much shine.

✳ Correct the hollow of the chin, if it is very prominent, using a concealer stick dotted on top of your regular foundation.

✳ To minimize a heavy jaw, try sweeping a little darker powder (faceshaper) along the jawline—make sure that you blend it in well.

✳ Disguise a double chin by brushing darker powder over the fleshy parts.

EYES

Eyes provide the perfect canvas for make-up
and offer the potential for creating many effects.
Remember, however: too much make-up, badly
applied, can distract and detract from the eyes
instead of flattering them. The value of eye make-up
is that it can subtly emphasize individual qualities
while playing down any imperfections. Most of us
would like to be able to achieve maximum impact
with a few deft strokes before we emerge to start
the day or in preparation for an evening out. The
following suggestions may help.

Almond oil makes a nourishing base for your eye make-up (blot the excess with a tissue to prevent your make-up from smearing).

Apply make-up around the eyes gently and evenly, on top of a light foundation and powder base. Make sure the foundation covers the temples and both the upper and lower eyelids.

Black eye liner tends to suit dark-eyed, dark-skinned women best, whereas brown and charcoal are more neutral, versatile shades.

When using eye liner, draw the line as close to your eyelashes as possible, top and bottom; if you like, gently smudge the line if you wish to soften the effect.

When choosing powder eyeshadow, steer clear of anything too obviously pearly or matte.

Keep your palette of eyeshadow colors fairly neutral—earth tones, smoky grays and browns, violets and heathery shades complement most eye colors and can be blended to create a natural effect.

When applying eyeshadow, apply the color thinly and gradually, darkest along the lid and at the outer corner of the eyes.

To apply mascara successfully, look down into a mirror and brush the lashes through slowly, from roots to tips. Start with the top side, then the underside of the upper lashes. Rest the brush on the outside of the lower lashes to give a light covering. Apply two or three thin coats for best results.

Almond oil is perfect for dissolving eye make-up and cleansing the eye area. If you wear a lot of eye make-up, cleanse twice, removing the excess oil by sweeping across the skin gently with a damp natural sponge or cotton wool pad.

CHEEKS

Make-up correctly applied to the cheeks can give you a healthy glow, and make the skin look even and smooth overall.

❀ Match skin tone with foundation: if the skin on your cheeks is dry, look for a creamy-textured formulation; an oil-free powder is more suitable for oily skin and enlarged pores.

❀ Apply foundation to the face using downward strokes with a damp make-up sponge, or just blend into areas of higher color with your fingers to even up skin tone. Don't forget to include neck, ears, and nostrils as well.

❀ For a natural glow, apply a touch of cream blusher to well-moisturized cheeks.

❧ To emphasize your cheekbones, load up a blusher brush with a small amount of color and blow off the excess. Sweep the brush across your cheekbones in the direction of—but short of—the hairline.

❧ Tie in your blusher color with your lipstick—if your lip color is "cool," your blusher color should be too.

❧ If you have full cheeks, try using a light application of a powder a shade darker than your foundation on the underside of cheekbones, blended out toward the ears—this adds definition.

❧ Foundation looks more finished when set with a very light dusting of loose translucent powder. Tip a small quantity into the palm of your hand, soak some up with a cotton wool pad, then apply. Remove any excess with a large brush or clean pad.

❧ Pressed translucent powder is a more practical choice when you are on the move.

LIPS

The general principle is that either your eyes or your mouth carry the day—never both. Putting on a slick of lipstick, even if the rest of your make-up is very low-key, can bring some much-needed color to the face and make it look "dressed" rather than "naked." While there is a limitless color range to choose from, this does not mean that every color will suit you—you will have to experiment. There is a knack to applying lipstick which is worth acquiring if you're interested in a professional finish and maximum staying power. Follow the basic principles overleaf for luscious-looking lips.

Once you have applied your moisturizer to the upper-lip area, apply a light wash of foundation with a damp sponge and set with a touch of powder. If you have darker blotches of skin, use a lighter foundation or concealer beneath the powder as a camouflage.

Lips need to be screened from potentially damaging ultraviolet rays and harsh winter weather, so look out for lipsticks with SPFs and other nourishing ingredients.

Match lipsticks to your skin tone rather than your clothes—plump for shades that flatter your complexion.

※ Try different formulations of lipstick to achieve the effect and level of coverage that you want, from a hint of sheer color to a deep, matte stain.

※ Always ring the changes: when you wear the same tried and tested lipsticks year after year, you can end up looking as though you are stuck in a time warp.

※ Look after your lips and keep them moist: even the most sophisticated lipstick formulation cannot make out-of-condition lips look sleek and luscious.

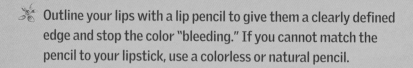 Outline your lips with a lip pencil to give them a clearly defined edge and stop the color "bleeding." If you cannot match the pencil to your lipstick, use a colorless or natural pencil.

A specially designed lip brush will help you to apply color with precision and make it stick. Blot each layer with a single-ply tissue and build up color until you are happy with the results. Brush a sprinkling of loose powder over the tissue to "fix."

JAWLINE

One of the most common make-up crimes is foundation that stops at the jawline, leaving a white ring around the neck! Don't make that mistake!

The skin tone of the neck is approximately the same as that on the inside of the forearms, so test foundation there to avoid a "tide mark" at the jawline when the shade is mismatched.

If you need a darker foundation for camouflaging purposes, apply color under the jawline and onto the neck and ears as well.

NAILS

Long, painted nails are not to everyone's taste—far better to keep nails neatly trimmed and well maintained, and to paint with a subtle, metallic color rather than glossy reds and pinks.

✻ Apply a base coat to fill in any irregularities on the surface of the nails. It will also provide a protective layer and prevent staining. Wipe off any drops that spill onto cuticles.

✻ Filling in the underside of the nail with a white nail pencil can make unpainted nails look prettier.

✻ Allow your nails to go unpainted for a few days every month so that they can "breathe."

✻ Beware of using dark colors, as any irregularities will be highlighted if the varnish is not well applied. Light, metallic colors are practical because pits and grooves are less conspicuous.

✻ Remove polish with acetone-free remover.

painting nails

Remove all traces of grease with soap and water before painting.

Make sure that the brush is not overloaded and that there is no polish on the stem.

Apply polish using three strokes—side, middle, side—starting with the little finger and working toward the thumb.

Allow polish to dry thoroughly before adding a second coat.

SEXUALITY

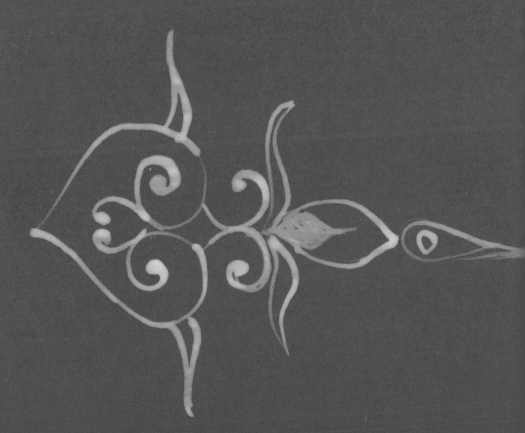

There are times in our lives when we can forget that we are sensual beings, and the pressures of modern life begin to take their toll on our sex drive. There are many natural ways in which you can boost your libido, and even just rediscover shared intimacy with your partner.

❧ St. John's wort is good at restoring lost interest in sex. It can lift mild depression within two weeks of starting a course. It can also help to get rid of anxiety, agitation, insomnia, and even headaches. Note: St. John's wort is not advised for women taking the oral contraceptive pill. Check with your doctor first.

❧ If you have a loss of sexual desire, take time to pamper yourself and remind yourself that you are a sensual creature: light candles, buy special bedlinen, play music, give yourself a manicure and pedicure, do your hair, and wear your best clothes.

❋ Take zinc to help maintain your sex drive, and evening primrose oil capsules, which contain the essential fatty acids your sex hormones need.

❋ To reinvigorate yourself after sex in the morning, drink some delicious almond milk. To make the milk, before going to bed, soak 10 raw almonds in water, then in the morning peel off the skins and blend them along with a pinch of nutmeg, saffron, and ginger, then add a cup of warm milk.

BHARTI VYAS SEXUALITY

aphrodisiac herbs

FOR MEN

Amla: This fruit has the highest proportion of vitamin C to be found in nature; clinical studies show that it increases the red blood cell count and reduces cholesterol. Dosage: 2 to 4 grams daily with meals.

Ashwagandha: This root of the winter cherry is well known in India as a semen promoter and is also used to treat infertility and impotence in men. It also helps to harmonise immune function, stabilize low blood pressure and regulate heartbeat. Dosage: 2 to 4 grams daily with milk or warm water.

Guggulu: The gum from a tree related to myrrh, guggulu reduces fat and toxins, is effective in treating arthritis, and is reputed to have aphrodisiac properties. Dosage: two 450mg tablets with meals, three times a day.

Haritaki: Clinical studies have shown that haritaki is effective against the herpes simplex virus, has antibacterial properties, increases the life of tissues and is even used to inhibit the HIV virus. Dosage: 2 to 5 grams per day.

FOR WOMEN

Kumari: Taken in fresh gel format this is renowned for its female rejuvenating properties, but should be avoided during pregnancy. In the USA it is often prescribed for disorders of the female reproductive system. You will need to take it daily for two menstrual cycles before observing results. Dosage: two tablespoons of gel twice a day.

Shatavari: This form of asparagus is an excellent daily supplement for all women. It is a phytoestrogen (naturally occurring), which helps to prevent the incidence of breast cancer and osteoporosis. For men it is believed to aid erectile tissue. Women need to use it regularly for a minimum of three menstrual cycles before seeing benefits. Dosage: 2 to 6 grams a day with meals.

If you feel tired and stressed in the evening, and sex seems like the last thing on your mind, have a relaxing hot bath, wash your own body gently, and then seduce your partner.

Stroking each other's skin in a non-sexual way is a natural therapy: if you massage and soothe each other's tired limbs you will maintain a precious familiarity with each other's bodies.

Rediscover intimate eye contact with your partner: lie or sit facing each other; hold hands and gaze into each other's eyes for a few minutes without talking, enjoying the feelings of intensity that arise through this process of reconnection.

MENOPAUSE

The menopause is the most significant symptom of advancing age in a woman's life. You are moving from a time of fertility to a time of reflection. For many women, such mental and physical changes are profoundly disturbing. For others, they are a blessed relief.

Your later years are a thing to be celebrated if you have looked after your health, body, and well-being. Ayurveda practitioners quote the following saying:

From the age of 0 to 16 you are a child
From the age of 16 to 70 you are young
From the age of 70 to 90 you are middle-aged
From the age of 90 to 120 you are old.

There is no reason why you shouldn't look and feel great in your menopause and beyond if you follow very simple rules about how to treat your body and mind.

minimizing symptoms

The secret to naturally minimizing hot sweats, headaches, and palpitations is to eat the food whose properties most closely mimic the effect of the body's natural hormones. Food rich in phytoestrogens include:

soya beans
linseed oil
green and yellow vegetables
ginseng
fennel
broccoli
rhubarb
celery

Top up your diet with a good multinutrient supplement, particularly one that has a mix of B-group vitamins.

❀ Increased irritability during menopause may be the result of low blood sugar levels—drink a glass of freshly squeezed orange juice, followed by a crisp-bread, slice of brown bread, or a banana.

❀ Menopausal anxiety tends to get better by itself—but cutting out alcohol and coffee will help.

❀ If you suffer from mood swings during the menopause, the best thing you can do is engage in regular energetic exercise. Even going for a walk on a daily basis can help to keep mood swings under control.

✳ Hot sweats can be relieved by cutting out stimulants such as tea, coffee, and alcohol, as well as foods like garlic, onion, and spices. Eat plenty of fruits and drink plenty of cold water.

✳ To relieve hot flashes, mix one teaspoon of organic sugar into a cup of pomegranate juice and eight drops of lime juice—you can drink this up to three times a day.

✳ Aromatherapy oils can help to relieve hot sweats: mix drops of chamomile or cypress into a sweet almond carrier oil.

❧ To avoid the risk of osteoporosis, take 1,500mg of calcium every day after the menopause, or drink an extra pint of skim or low-fat milk every day.

❧ Natural progesterone cream is extracted from wild yams and can help prevent osteoporosis. Applied regularly onto a part of the body where the skin is thin (e.g. inner arm) it is also a good way to enhance mood and general well-being.

WEIGHT GAIN DURING MENOPAUSE

The metabolic rate alters around the time of menopause,
so rather than trying to eat less, increase your metabolic rate
by exercising more. Swimming, walking, and golf are all excellent
gentle pursuits to help keep you in trim.

Falling hormone levels during the menopause may affect
your hunger—even though you've just eaten you still feel
hungry. Drink a glass of fizzy water mixed with some lemon,
or clean your teeth to signal to your stomach that no more
food is forthcoming.

FACT

DURING MENOPAUSE, THERE ARE MANY HORMONE CHANGES HAPPENING IN THE BODY—
JUST THE SAME AS DURING ADOLESCENCE, BUT WITH THE ADDITION OF 45 YEARS OF
ABUSE ON TOP! HENCE MANY WOMEN FIND IT DIFFICULT TO LOSE WEIGHT AS EASILY AS
THEY DID WHEN THEY WERE YOUNGER—FATTY TISSUES SPREAD ACROSS THE STOMACH
AND SKIN, AND THE SKIN IS NO LONGER ELASTIC ENOUGH TO SPRING BACK AGAIN.
HOWEVER, IF YOU TAKE THE TIME WHEN APPROACHING MENOPAUSE TO KEEP A CHECK ON
YOUR FOOD INTAKE, GENERAL HEALTH, AND WELL-BEING, AND EXERCISE REGULARLY,
YOU CAN AVOID THIS PROBLEM WITHOUT HAVING TO ADHERE TO A STRICT DIET.

- To trick your mid-life fat cells, ditch the diets for good, and eat five or six small meals a day.

- In any healthy diet, but especially when approaching menopause, increase your fiber intake, cut down on the amount of salt in your diet, and avoid an excess of fatty foods.

SEX

Sex is really is good for you—according to recent research, women who are approaching menopause and still having sex weekly, experience fewer hot sweats than those who are not sexually active.

Sex is a great form of exercise, and helps to relieve stress and tension. So enjoy yourself!

index

acknowledgments

I would like to dedicate this book to all my clients and to the many readers of my books who have gained control of their health and well-being. A huge thanks to my loving family who have always worked tirelessly and supported me unconditionally. My husband Raja, my two precious daughters Shailu and Priti, my grandchildren Anjali, Neha, Saajan ,and Serena, and my sons-in-law Bharath and Parag.

I would also like to thank the team at my holistic center, in particular Magda Waldron and Rakesh Shah. A special thanks to Caroline Shott, my literary agent, who has been a tremendous support to me. To Gail Rebuck and her team at Random House who have worked with such enthusiasm and commitment to produce this fantastic book: to Fiona MacIntyre, Carey Smith, Eileen Campbell, Sarah Lavelle, Clare Lawler, and Caroline Newbury my sincere appreciation and thanks. To the Skin Wisdom Team at Tesco's, especially Kari Daniels, Kerry Robinson, Jacqueline Grattan, Vanessa Campbell, Helen Massey, Clare Barr, and Jane Beechey and her PR team at BMA. To everyone at the Federation of Holistic Therapists (FHT), including Mr. Sharp, Jacqueline Palmer, and Colin Young, especially to all those who have supported all my professional work and principles. Also thanks to Heather Mole and her team at VTCT. To Heather Ewing and her fabulous team at Centre Parcs. To Baby Mathew from the fantastic Somatheeram Ayurvedic Resort in Trivendrum, India.

Last, but definitely not least, to my dear friend the late Dr. Ginsberg, who was always a wealth of knowledge to me.